Everyone's Guide to
OUTPATIENT
SURGERY

◆

JAMES MACHO MD
AND GREG CABLE

A Somerville House Book

◆

Andrews and McMeel
A Universal Press Syndicate Company
Kansas City

For information, please write to:
Andrews and McMeel,
a Universal Press Syndicate Company,
4900 Main Street,
Kansas City, Missouri 64112

Library of Congress Cagaloging-in-Publication Data

Everyone's guide to outpatient surgery / [edited by] James Macho and
  Greg Cable.
      p.   cm.
      "A Somerville House book".
      Includes bibliographical references and index.
      ISBN 0-8362-2421-3
      1. Ambulatory surgery—Popular works.   I. Macho, James.
II. Cable, Greg, 1946- .
RD110.E885 1994
617'.024—dc20

                                        94-17957
                                           CIP

hc

Printed in the United States of America

Book Design by Falcom Design and Communications Inc.
Edited by Ruth Chernia

Produced by Somerville House Books Limited
        3080 Yonge Street, Suite 5000
        Toronto, Ontario
        M4N 3N1

To my wife, Rosaire
and
to my children, Jennifer and James, Jr.
JM

In memory of Dr. John Hay. Great joy.
GC

CONTENTS

———◇———

15. Orthopedic Surgery 122

16. Hand Surgery 132

ACKNOWLEDGEMENTS

When I undertook this project, I did not realize the amount of time and effort that would be necessary to bring *Everyone's Guide to Outpatient Surgery* to completion. This book would not have been possible without the support, help and encouragement of many people.

I am particularly thankful to have worked with Greg Cable, my co-writer. With contributing authors demanding that not a single word in their chapters be changed, he was successfully able to modify many highly technical and complex manuscripts in order to make them clear and easily understood by the general public. I have the utmost respect for his competence and sense of humor.

I would like to thank my contributing authors for taking the time out of their busy practices to share their knowledge and expertise in this book. These authors were chosen not only because of their reputations as superb clinicians but even more so because of their particular talents as outstanding teachers. Their strong commitment to patient education was the driving force behind this book.

I wish to acknowledge the artistic contributions of the medical illustrator, Kam Yu. His illustrations are very clear and they complement the text well.

I am grateful to Jane Somerville for supporting the concept of a book on Outpatient Surgery and for providing the opportunity for its creation. I am thankful to her, Patrick Crean and the others at Somerville House for their continued encouragement along the way.

I extend warm thanks to Ruth Chernia, my managing editor, for her extraordinary efforts in bringing this book to completion. I am sure that it was a new experience for her to work on a book written primarily by surgeons. Her exceptional patience was greatly appreciated when deadlines passed without the submission of manuscripts due to emergencies and the other unexpected demands that I and my colleagues face on a regular basis. Nevertheless, her persistence and concern never wavered. Her willingness to learn the art of file exchange by modem was also greatly appreciated.

I would like to extend my grateful appreciation to my American publisher at Andrews and McMeel.

I extend particular thanks to Ernest Rosenbaum, MD, the co-author of *Everyone's Guide to Cancer Therapy*. His enthusiasm and support convinced me to take on this project. I am grateful that he introduced me to the publishers at Somerville House. I am also very grateful for the time he took in reviewing the entire book and providing invaluable advice and criticism.

I would like to thank Marcia Evans, CNRA, for the suggestions and information that she provided for the Anesthesia chapter while we were waiting for our respective flights at the Washington, D.C.-Dulles International Airport.

I would like to offer my most special and sincere thanks to my wife Rosaire and to my children. They had to contend with more than the usual number of canceled plans and weekends without me due to "the book." I am particularly grateful to my wife for her authorship of two chapters and for her excellent advice and suggestions on the other parts of the book. Her career as a nursing educator has been temporarily "on hold" while she devotes the majority of her time to our children. I am also thankful for her invaluable administrative and technical assistance. I regret the many times that she had to take the dreaded telephone calls from editors who were very concerned about whether a particular deadline would be met.

Finally, I would like to thank my patients. Their trust and confidence has made my profession very rewarding. By sharing their concerns with me, they suggested the need for this book. I am grateful to those patients who reviewed the early chapters and made important suggestions. I would like to recognize the willingness of most patients and their families to become active partners in the delivery of their surgical care. I feel strongly that this has been primarily responsible for the growth and success of outpatient surgery.

James R. Macho, MD, FACS
San Francisco, California 1994

FOREWORD

Orlo H. Clark, MD

———————◇———————

For many years, people have been fascinated about medicine and medical science. This has never been more evident than today when medical topics are reported daily in the media.

This timely book by James R. Macho, MD, and co-authors, is a comprehensive volume for patients and health professionals. It provides accurate information to patients and their families about what to expect, what to ask, and what they should know when scheduled for an outpatient surgical procedure. Dr. Macho has organized a formidable group of medical professionals, primarily faculty at the University of California, San Francisco/Mount Zion Medical Center, who are experts in their respective specialties of surgery or are nurses who are experienced in outpatient surgical units.

Today, more and more operations are performed in outpatient surgical units rather than as inpatient procedures. Such a shift is due to advances in anesthesia, surgical techniques, medications, and nursing care. Outpatient surgery is also more cost effective and is often less frightening and produces less anxiety for patients. As well, patients appear to recover more quickly.

The book is comprehensive. There are chapters about most of the surgical techniques that are done by general surgeons, plastic surgeons, and dermatologists as well as peripheral vascular surgeons, proctologists, ophthalmologists, otolaryngologists, orthopedists, hand surgeons, gynecologists, and urologists.

Illustrations have been used selectively to clarify the anatomy and procedures. Overall, this text will help inform patients and give them sufficient facts to ask informed questions and to select an experienced surgeon.

This volume should be in every library and every doctor's office.

CONTRIBUTORS

James Macho, MD, FACS
Assistant Clinical Professor of Surgery, University of California, San Francisco, School of Medicine.

Attending Surgeon and Director of Surgical Critical Care, University of California, San Francisco/Mt. Zion Medical Center.

Fellow, American College of Surgeons, Fellow, American College of Chest Physicians and member of the Association for Surgical Education.

James R. Macho received his medical degree from the Harvard Medical School. He completed a Residency in General Surgery and a Fellowship in Critical Care Medicine at the University of California, San Francisco.

In addition to his surgical practice and patient care activities, Dr. Macho teaches at the UCSF School of Medicine and in the UCSF Surgical Residency Program. He is the Director of the UCSF surgical clerkship for third year medical students and has won several awards for excellence in teaching. He has lectured extensively at regional and national surgical conferences and has authored and co-authored many articles and book chapters dealing with surgery and surgical critical care. He is currently working on a textbook of outpatient surgery.

Dr. Malin Roy Dollinger's lifelong dedication to patient education and the field of oncology has included a research post at the Memorial Sloan Kettering Cancer Center in New York as well as a post as Director of Medical Oncology at Harbor General Hospital/ UCLA Medical Center in Los Angeles. He lectures extensively about cancer and is co-author of *Everyone's Guide to Cancer Therapy*, in this same series.

Dr. Ernest H. Rosenbaum is also a co-author of *Everyone's Guide to Cancer Therapy* and is a practicing oncologist in San Francisco at Mt. Zion Medical Center of UCSF. A co-founder of the Northern California Academy of Clinical Oncology, Dr. Rosenbaum has received Honorable Mention from the American Medical Writers Association for Excellence in Medical Publications for *A Comprehensive Guide for Cancer Patients and Their Families.*

Greg Cable has been a writer and editor since 1970; he has co-authored several books including *Everyone's Guide to Cancer Therapy* and *Catch: A Major League Life*, the best-selling autobiography of former Toronto Blue Jays catcher Ernie Whitt.

Robert Allen, MD, FACS
Clinical Professor of Surgery
University of California, San Francisco, CA

Jennifer F. Bock, MD
Chief Resident in Otolaryngology
University of California,
San Francisco, CA

Damien Bolton, MD
Department of Urology
UCSF/Mt. Zion Medical Center,
San Francisco, CA

Jeannette S. Brown, MD
Assistant Professor of Obstetrics &
Gynecology
University of California, San Francisco, CA

F. Charles Brunicardi, MD, FACS
Assistant Professor of Surgery
University of California,
Los Angeles, CA

David Chang, MD, FACS
Opthalmologic Surgery
Palo Alto, CA

Orlo H. Clark, MD
Professor and Vice-chair of Surgery
University of California School of Medicine,
San Francisco, CA
President, International Association of
Endocrine Surgeons
Chief of Surgery, UCSF/Mt. Zion
Medical Center, San Francisco, CA

Robert S. Dorian, MD
Department of Anesthesia
St. Barnabas Hospital,
Livingston, NJ

Issa Eshima, MD
Assistant Professor of Plastic and
Reconstructive Surgery
University of California, San Francisco, CA

Stanley Leong, MD, FACS
Director, UCSF/Mt. Zion Breast Care Center
Associate Professor of Surgery
University of California, San Francisco, CA

David W. Lowenberg, MD
Assistant Clinical Professor Department
of Orthopedic Surgery
University of California, San Francisco, CA

James R. Macho, MD, FACS
Director of Surgical Critical Care
UCSF/Mt. Zion Medical Center
Assistant Professor of Surgery
University of California, San Francisco, CA

Lynne Macho, RN
Scripps Memorial Hospital
La Jolla, CA

Rosaire F. Macho, RN, BSN
Principal, Slide Effects
Mill Valley, CA

Robert Markison, MD, FACS
Associate Clinical Professor of Surgery
University of California, San Francisco, CA

Jeffrey Pearl, MD, FACS
Director, Vascular Access Service
UCSF/Mt. Zion Medical Center
Associate Clinical Professor of Surgery
University of California,
San Francisco, CA

Loie Sauer, MD, FACS
Vascular and General Surgery
Santa Rosa, CA

William P. Schecter, MD, FACS
Chief of Surgery,
San Francisco General Hospital
Associate Clinical Professor of Surgery
University of California,
San Francisco, CA

Mark I. Singer, MD
Chief of Otolaryngology and Head and
Neck Surgery
UCSF/Mt. Zion Medical Center
Professor of Otolaryngology
University of California, San Francisco
Chief of Otolaryngology and Head and
Neck Surgery
UCSF/Mt. Zion Medical Center,
San Francisco, CA

Alan Siperstein, MD, FACS
Assistant Professor of Surgery
University of California,
San Francisco, CA

Marshall Stoller, MD
Assistant Professor of Surgery
University of California,
San Francisco, CA

1
OUTPATIENT SURGERY AND THE CHANGING FACE OF HEALTH CARE

James R. Macho, MD, FACS

———◇———

Outpatient surgery is the common term for the situation where a patient arrives at a surgical suite in the morning, undergoes surgery, has a brief recovery, then goes home the same day. It is sometimes called ambulatory surgery or day surgery.

This type of surgery has increased dramatically in the past 15 years. More than half of all surgical procedures performed in the United States are now being done on an outpatient basis. More than 200 procedures can now be performed this way.

This trend toward more outpatient surgery has proven to be of great benefit to patients. Surgery used to be tremendously disruptive for a patient. Consider the experience you would have had as recently as 1980 with the experience you will have today.

The Days of Extended Hospitalization
If you had developed an inguinal hernia only a decade or so ago, you would have been admitted to the hospital the day before the scheduled surgery.

After providing information and filling out numerous forms, you would have been taken to a room on the surgical ward and asked to change into a hospital gown. Technicians would have come to your room to draw blood samples for laboratory tests and possibly to perform an electrocardiogram. If a chest x-ray was required, people from the radiology department would have come to escort you to the x-ray room.

During the afternoon, you would have been seen by a physician who would perform a complete history and physical examination. You would then be visited by the anesthesiologist for another examination and a chat about the proposed method of anesthesia.

The surgeon would have come to give you a detailed description of the procedure and answer any questions. If the surgeon came during visiting hours, your family might also have participated in the discussion. If he or she came at some other time, your family might never have seen the surgeon at all.

You would have then had the opportunity to sleep in an uncomfortable hospital bed, often on a ward that was noisy and not conducive to a restful sleep.

The following morning you would have been taken to one of the main operating rooms in the surgical suite. Many other procedures would be in progress in adjacent operating rooms, perhaps open heart surgery, brain surgery or complex cancer operations. If emergencies occurred, your relatively minor surgery could have been delayed or even canceled.

When the operation was completed, you would have been transferred to the recovery room for several hours, before returning to the surgery ward. To relieve any pain, you would usually have been given narcotics by injection, which would be effective but would also make you drowsy. You would not have been given anything to eat or drink on the day of surgery, being maintained with fluids given intravenously.

Over two to three days, you would have been weaned from the injections and put on oral pain medications. Gradually, you would have been given solid foods and have been allowed to walk around the ward. Finally, you would have been discharged.

This three- to four-day stay in the hospital would likely have resulted in major inconveniences. You might have shared a room with a seriously ill patient having frequent visits from doctors and nurses that would have interrupted your sleep. Removed from your familiar surroundings and with limited access to your family because of rigid visiting hours, you would not have been able to use your time in the hospital for any productive activities. Most of your time would have been spent waiting for someone or for something to happen.

It is also possible that you would have been at some slight risk of developing an infection after surgery since other patients on the ward may have had infections with virulent strains of hospital bacteria.

What Happens Now If you are having an inguinal hernia repaired today, you will sleep in your own bed the night before surgery and wake up early to go to an outpatient surgery center. Your history, physical examination and lab and other tests will have been completed the week before. All admission forms will have been filled out and approved during the same period. You will have discussed the procedure with your surgeon during a preoperative visit and all your questions will have been answered. Your family will have also had the chance to speak with the surgeon during a preoperative visit.

On arrival at the ambulatory surgery suite, you'll be greeted by staff who deal exclusively with these and similar procedures. You will know that your surgery will proceed close to the scheduled time since emergency procedures won't affect the schedule.

Once the operation is done, the surgeon or anesthetist will inject a long-acting local anesthetic in the area of the incision. After transfer to the recovery room, you will recover rapidly from the anesthetic and be ready for transfer to the ambulatory surgery suite within 60 to 90 minutes. There, you will be closely watched and carefully evaluated. Within an hour, you might be given liquids to drink. After a visit from the surgeon, you will be allowed to return home.

On discharge, you will be provided with oral pain medications and detailed instructions. If you have questions or problems, you can contact your surgeon, although in most cases that won't be necessary.

On the night of surgery, you can sleep in your own bed and wake up in the morning in your own home.

SURGERY TODAY

The difference between the above two scenarios indicates one major reason why outpatient surgery is becoming more common: patients enthusiastically prefer it to inpatient surgery.

But when the concept was introduced, patients and physicians resisted it. The resistance was based mainly on concerns about safety. Doctors worried about problems and complications when their patients weren't being constantly watched by nurses or other medical professionals. Patients worried about something bad happening without a medical safety net close by.

Experience soon demonstrated, however, that when patients are carefully selected, outpatient surgery is as safe as inpatient surgery. That safety comes in part from the dramatic advances in the field of surgery over the past few years.

About 150 years ago, in the days before anesthesia, surgery was called "the brutal craft." The best surgeon was the one who worked fastest. Some surgeons prided themselves on being able to amputate a leg in 20 seconds. The discovery of anesthesia in the 1860s changed surgery dramatically. Within 10 years, appendectomies were being performed. Within 20 years, gallbladders and other abdominal organs were being treated surgically. The range of procedures continued to expand throughout this century, with a trend to more and more complex operations, such as open heart surgery.

Since the 1970s, however, for a great number of reasons, many operations have become *less* complex.

Greater Knowledge Medical research has resulted in major new developments in surgery and anesthesia. Advances in preoperative management, newer antibiotics and less-invasive surgical techniques allow more procedures to be performed on an outpatient basis. Minimally invasive surgery performed via the laparoscope offers the advantages of tiny scars, less postoperative pain and a more rapid return to full activity. Newer anesthetics have reduced postoperative nausea and drowsiness. New oral analgesic medications allow for excellent postoperative pain control without the need for injections. With further advances, it is likely that many procedures will be performed in the outpatient setting.

Imaging Techniques Twenty years ago surgeons regularly performed an operation called an exploratory laparotomy. This was done when the doctor couldn't figure out exactly what was wrong in the patient's belly. The abdomen would

be cut open so the surgeon could look around to discover the true nature of the problem. That kind of operation is almost never performed today, except in cases of trauma such as a car accident.

Now, when surgeons operate they usually know exactly what the problem is and what the extent of the problem is. Every operation can be very well planned out and the scope of the procedure can be narrowed considerably.

Imaging techniques such as computerized tomography (CT) and magnetic resonance imaging (MRI) have played a big part in this change. A CT scan is in a sense a radiologic laparotomy because all the organs can be seen and evaluated. CT lets a surgeon localize the abnormal area, and in many cases a needle can be put into the belly with CT guidance to do a biopsy. For example, if the surgeon sees an abnormal spot in the liver, she or he can go in and remove a piece of the suspicious tissue to find out whether it is cancerous. These techniques can be used with almost all the abdominal organs.

Advances in Surgical Technology With the development of new techniques, procedures that once required a one-week hospital admission and up to six months of disability are now performed on an outpatient basis with only a week before a patient may return to regular activity.

Many procedures that used to involve major abdominal incisions are now performed using laparoscopic techniques. In this approach, a small incision is made near the navel. A telescope with a tiny video camera is inserted through this incision. Additional instruments are then inserted through other small incisions. Rather than leaving a large wound, patients have several tiny wounds that require only Band-Aids.

Similar procedures are now used for what formerly were major operations in gynecology and urology. Orthopedic surgeons operate inside joints with telescopes called arthroscopes. Polyps in the colon are removed with an endoscope and other specialized instruments, thereby eliminating the need for major abdominal surgery.

Changes in Surgical Technique
Modifications of standard surgical procedures have made surgery easier and minimized postoperative pain. What has particularly improved over the past 15 years is the safety and the extent of scarring. Large incisions used to be the norm even for relatively simple operations like hernia repairs. Today, incisions are much smaller, which means the patient is more comfortable and is left with a smaller scar.

Improved Anesthesia and Pain Control
The need for general anesthesia was once thought to disqualify a patient for outpatient surgery. Now, general anesthesia is used in more than half of outpatient surgery cases. Newer anesthetic agents are fast acting, meaning that anesthesia is induced rapidly and easily and the recovery time is shorter. These new agents also eliminate many problems with nausea and vomiting.

The injection of long-acting local anesthetics into incisions and the use of highly effective and safe oral medications have greatly reduced pain after an operation.

THE ADVANTAGES OF OUTPATIENT SURGERY
Outpatient surgery benefits everyone in the health care system—patients, doctors, nurses, administrators and other health care professionals. There are many advantages.

Less Patient Anxiety and Disruption
When presented with the option, most people prefer to have their surgery on an outpatient basis.
◆ By staying out of the hospital, patients are subjected to much less disruption of their home life and lose less time from work or school.
◆ When outpatient surgery is performed in a specialized center, there is generally much less of a wait than if the surgery was performed in a regular hospital operating room.
◆ A shorter waiting time can result in less preoperative anxiety and disability.

Quality Care Outpatient surgery staff are highly skilled at the smaller number of procedures.
◆ Many studies have shown that the outcome from outpatient surgery is the same as that from inpatient surgery and that the safety record is almost identical.

Fewer Infections Several studies have shown that people undergoing outpatient surgery have fewer postoperative infections, probably because they are not exposed to the bacteria normally present on hospital wards.
◆ In those rare cases when outpatient surgical patients do develop infections, they are usually infected with organisms found in the home. They may already have defenses against these bacteria and can often fight off the infections quite readily. If treatment is required, these "home-grown" bacteria are usually susceptible to standard antibiotics.

Efficiency Outpatient surgery provides great benefits for the surgical team.
◆ With outpatient surgery, the time between operations may be as little as 15 minutes. Nothing spills on the floor or the operating table, and very little clean-up is required.
◆ The starting times for surgical procedures are reliably predicted. Realistic and accurate scheduling of cases allows a surgeon to use his or her time more

effectively. The backlog of surgical cases is reduced and other scheduled activities are not disrupted when surgery is delayed or postponed.

◆ Equipment can be standardized.

◆ The similarity of cases allows the nursing staff to become very knowledgeable. As efficiency is achieved, more time can be spent with patients in education activities. Nurses find their work much more satisfying when they are performing these types of activities rather than administrative tasks.

Reduced Costs It's no secret that the cost of health care has been increasing dramatically in this country, mostly because of hospital costs. Hospitals are expensive institutions to run, and this fact helped spur the trend toward shorter hospital stays. That in turn spurred the trend to more surgical procedures being performed without any hospital stay at all.

There is no question that outpatient surgery reduces medical costs substantially.

◆ Patients often require fewer expensive preoperative diagnostic tests. When the tests are obtained outside of the hospital, they can usually be performed much more economically.

◆ Hospital inpatient services are expensive, and the average hospital room costs $800 to $1,000 a day. Much of this cost pays for round-the-clock nursing and other supportive care for all patients. People with great expertise are on call at all times. With outpatient procedures, the availability of people with expertise is maintained, but the cost is borne only by those patients who need their services.

◆ Outpatient operating rooms are maintained much more economically than regular hospital operating rooms. Expensive and highly specialized equipment is not required. Overhead is much lower, since these operating rooms are not staffed 24 hours a day.

◆ Depending on whether the procedure is done in a hospital outpatient center or a free-standing facility, the cost of outpatient surgery is generally 25 to 50 percent less than inpatient surgery—with identical safety and effectiveness.

DISADVANTAGES OF OUTPATIENT SURGERY

Less Access to Services The obvious disadvantage is the decreased level of access to inpatient services. With careful selection of patients, however, this is usually not a problem because very few patients will need these services.

◆ It has been estimated that one of every 100 patients scheduled for outpatient surgery will require hospital admission. In most cases, the reason for admission is postoperative nausea and vomiting or postoperative pain not relieved by oral pain medications. It is extremely rare for a serious problem to develop, though all outpatient surgery centers have provisions for such situations.

◆ If the outpatient surgery suite is in a hospital, it is generally a simple matter of arranging for a hospital room and an overnight stay. In cases where the patient is undergoing surgery at a separate outpatient surgery facility, transport to a hospital will be required.

Postoperative Complications One reason patients used to be kept in the hospital for several days was concern that problems could develop after surgery. But even in those days, few people developed complications, and it was easy to recognize soon after surgery which ones were likely to have them.

The potential of postoperative complications occurring while the patient is at home may be minimized by careful patient selection.

◆ Even if the risk of a complication is only slightly increased, the surgeon will recommend that the patient be admitted to the hospital and the operation be performed in the hospital's regular operating rooms.

♦ With appropriate education, patients and their families can recognize complications and quickly contact their surgeon for advice. Early recognition and timely treatment usually result in a successful outcome.

Greater Patient Responsibility Leaving aside the disruption to daily life, surgery used to be rather convenient for patients. Everything was done for them and usually in a first-class manner. Now patients have to bear much more responsibility for their own care. In many cases, family and friends also have to take on some significant responsibilities.

♦ Patients are given a checklist of all the places they have to go before their surgery. They will usually have to spend a good part of a day stopping for lab tests or visiting the x-ray department, for example. The system is efficient, but there are many bases to cover. Unfortunately, the journey usually involves the frustrations of waiting at each stop.

♦ After the operation, patients and their families have to be responsible for managing dressings, inspecting wounds and providing medications.

♦ Having to take responsibility need not be a disadvantage, however. In most cases, patients and their families feel it is a small price to pay for the major advantage of staying out of the hospital.

YOUR ROLE AS AN OUTPATIENT

As an outpatient, you are a more active participant in your health maintenance and care.

Medical treatment is a team effort. And if you are going to work together with doctors, nurses, technicians and other specialists to make surgery or any other treatment a successful and non-threatening experience, you as a patient have to become informed.

Having surgery, whether as an inpatient or outpatient, can be a stressful time for you and the people around you. But if you approach your surgery armed with information about what you can expect before, during and after your operation, you will have the knowledge and confidence you need to make your surgery a more positive experience.

2
YOUR SURGEON AND THE DECISION TO HAVE SURGERY

James R. Macho, MD, FACS

———————◇———————

If you are consulting a surgeon, it is likely that your regular physician has identified a condition that can be cured or at least relieved by surgery. Your physician may have given you the name of a surgeon to contact or may have made an appointment for you. Or your physician may have left the choice of a surgeon entirely up to you.

Whatever the options you are offered, ultimately it is your decision both to proceed with the surgery and to use the services of a particular surgeon. Those decisions can be made only after an initial consultation where you will have the chance to discuss the procedure and to find out whether you trust and feel comfortable with the surgeon.

As soon as you are referred to a surgeon, you enter a world that may well be outside your normal experience with the health care system. Surgeons have the reputation within and beyond the medical community of being a little bit different, and that is, in fact, the case—for many reasons.

When you are sick, your medical doctor might try various antibiotics or other medications to help you overcome disease. If these medications don't work, your doctor will try something else or even switch to some other form of treatment altogether. Very rarely is any harm done by giving ineffective medication the first time around.

Surgery, on the other hand, is irrevocable. For the most part, once a surgeon has done something, he or she cannot go back and undo it.

Having surgery is a big step. When you see a surgeon, you are putting your well-being and, indeed, your very life into the hands of a stranger. Who is this person, and what are the surgeon's qualifications for having such a profound influence on your life?

A SURGEON'S TRAINING

As with any other medical specialty, becoming a surgeon requires many years of education beyond medical school. To become a general surgeon, the minimum period is usually five years of clinical training as a hospital resident. Some surgical specialties may require seven to 10 years of training.

Residency The first year after medical school is spent as a medical intern, taking care of patients on hospital wards before and after surgery. During this year, the surgeon in training may not have much of an opportunity to take part in operations, although he or she observes many procedures and may have the chance to put in some stitches or tie a few knots.

Over the next few years, the resident gradually takes on greater responsibilities in the operating room, performing more and more of the surgical procedure. In the last year of training as a chief resident, he or she performs entire operations under the close supervision of a senior surgeon.

Further Specialization Physicians specializing in orthopedic, pediatric, vascular and plastic surgery or in fields such as gynecology, urology and ophthalmology often complete their first year of residency with general surgery residents and then go on to complete three or four years of additional training in their specific area.

Certification After the five or more years of surgical training, the surgeon goes into practice and begins to operate independently. Within the first year, a hospital requires that the surgeon take two examinations to become certified by the American Board of Surgery. Certification by the Board means that the surgeon has met exacting standards of education and practice.

The first examination is a day-long written test to answer more than a thousand extremely difficult questions about all areas of surgery. Success in this exam qualifies the surgeon to take the certifying examination. This involves responding to clinical scenarios presented by a panel of doctors.

The certification is valid for 10 years, after which the surgeon's practice and credentials are re-examined during a recertification process. This ensures that the surgeon has kept abreast of new surgical thinking and advanced techniques and continues to practice according to the American Board of Surgery's exacting standards.

The College of Surgeons During the year after certification, the surgeon records the details of all operations and, at the end of the year, can apply to become a Fellow of the American College of Surgeons. This puts the surgeon's practice under extreme scrutiny. The surgeon is closely questioned on such matters as preoperative and postoperative diagnoses, procedures and pathologies for all operations performed.

About 75 percent of American surgeons are Fellows of the College.

Individual Surgical Style Board certification and membership in the College indicate that the surgeon has demonstrated specialized knowledge and skill of a very high standard. But this does not mean that every surgeon will perform a particular procedure in exactly the same way. Surgery is an art as well as a science.

Surgical residents usually work with 30 or 40 surgeons and eventually develop their own style. In practice, some surgeons work very fast, some work more slowly. Surgeons make incisions in various ways, may use somewhat different instruments or follow different steps to complete a particular procedure and then may close the wound with various types of sutures or surgical staples.

The point to remember is that there are different ways of doing things. If one surgeon makes a larger incision than another, the surgeon making the larger incision has not done something wrong. There is room in the profession for personal style and preference based on training and experience.

THE SURGEON'S ROLE

There is a popular stereotype of a surgeon as a "hired gun" who comes into a case at the last minute, does all the necessary cutting and sewing, then turns the patient back to the medical doctor to take care of everything else.

Today, surgeons are closely involved with their patients before and after an operation, as well as in the operating room. From the first consultation, your surgeon will perform many tasks.

Evaluate Your Condition When a physician refers you for evaluation, the surgeon will usually see you in her or his office. The surgeon will take your complete history, review whatever studies your physician has performed, such as blood tests or x-rays, and conduct an examination.

Some people are surprised that the surgeon performs a complete physical examination, thinking that she or he is just duplicating what the medical doctor has already done. Surgeons, however, may be looking for other things that could be important in performing the operation. In some cases, the surgeon's examination will be more thorough than the medical doctor's.

During this consultation, the surgeon will make a decision about the appropriateness of surgery for your problem. This opinion will be told to you and, in a letter that may be dictated in your presence, to the referring physician.

Explain the Procedure and Answer Questions The surgeon will explain, with illustrations, what he or she proposes to do and will outline the benefits, discuss alternative forms of treatment and explore any surgical options, risks, complications and consequences. The decision to have surgery always involves a balance of these factors.

The surgeon will also answer any questions or talk about any concerns you might have.

Deal with Your Insurance Company In any surgeon's office in the United States, several hours of staff time and perhaps an hour of the surgeon's time each day are spent meeting the information needs of insurance companies. Insurance companies today are very demanding. They question more procedures and tend to allow less time in the hospital, which is one of the forces driving the growth of outpatient surgery.

There are many insurance companies, and they each have their own ways of operating. At one end of the spectrum, a company may have a book of reasons why an operation should be done. If the surgeon's information matches up, permission to do the operation is speedily given. At the opposite end, some companies require in all cases that the surgeon call up the company's own doctor and explain in great detail why a procedure is necessary and what hospitalization, tests and expenses are anticipated. Other companies want to see all documentation such as x-rays or ultrasound reports before giving their approval.

Schedule the Surgery The surgeon's office will schedule the surgery and make arrangements for any tests or examinations that might be required. The office staff will give you a complete list of what you will have to do to prepare for the operation (*see* Chapter 3).

Plan for Anesthesia There are usually three possibilities for anesthetic: local, regional and general (*see* Chapter 5). The surgeon will discuss these alternatives with you at the initial meeting and will usually recommend one method as the most appropriate for your particular procedure.

◆ If only a local anesthetic is needed, the surgeon will usually give the injection and no anesthesiologist will be involved.

◆ Some medical factors, such as obesity or a history of heart or lung disease, might indicate the wisdom of having an anesthesiologist standing by just in case the local doesn't work as well as it should. In the stand-by situation, the anesthesiologist will give you intravenous sedation and will be available to perform other services if the operation becomes more complicated than expected.

◆ For procedures where general or regional anesthesia is necessary, the anesthesiologist will see you beforehand to evaluate your condition and give an opinion about whether any other tests are needed before going ahead with the operation.

Perform the Operation Except for very minor procedures, there are always two physicians in the operating room, along with the rest of the medical team. For many surgical procedures, more than two hands are required. The primary surgeon controls the steps and the way things are done, which is the most important part of the operation. The assistant surgeon performs various tasks as directed by the primary surgeon.

Sometimes the assisting surgeon is a resident. Some patients are concerned about a resident being involved in the surgery. A resident may handle some technical aspects of the procedure, including some of the cutting and sewing, but the critical thinking and planning are always done by your surgeon.

Manage Postoperative Pain After your operation, you will need some means of relieving pain. Some people do not want to take any pain medication, either because of personal standards of keeping a "stiff upper lip" or because they have an unwarranted fear of becoming addicted to painkillers. But relief from pain is important. You will need to be relatively pain-free so you can take deep breaths, cough and walk around, all of which are necessary to promote healing.

Not taking pain medication might prove harmful. If you can't take deep breaths because of the pain, it is possible that portions of your lung will collapse. This can quickly lead to pneumonia and breathing difficulties. In an extreme case, a patient might require intensive care and mechanical ventilation.

Your surgeon, rather than your regular physician, should be in charge of the program to manage postoperative pain. The surgeon will want to know if you need extra pain medication, because this could indicate a problem. Unexpected severe pain may indicate a collection of blood (hematoma) putting pressure on a nerve. Increasing pain three days after the operation may mean that an infection is developing or some other complication is in process.

The surgeon will also want to evaluate the type of medication you take. A common and moderately strong pain medication such as codeine, for example, causes constipation. If you are constipated, you will likely strain during bowel movements, which could put pressure or tension on your incision or the surgical repair. If you are having more pain than expected, the surgeon will prescribe medications that are non-constipating or make sure you are taking other medications such as stool softeners to relieve the constipation.

Follow Up Your surgeon will be closely involved with any follow-up procedures necessary after the operation. With very simple procedures, follow-up may involve only removing staples or stitches or examining your incision for evidence of infection or other problems.

With more complex procedures, you may be required to see your surgeon several times after the operation and you may have to undergo blood or other tests to make sure the operation was successful.

IS OUTPATIENT SURGERY RIGHT FOR YOU?

Once the surgeon concludes that surgery is appropriate, the next decision she or he has to make is whether you can have the procedure on an outpatient basis. Many procedures lend themselves to outpatient surgery, but there is a limit to what can be done. This type of surgery is not suitable for all procedures nor for all patients. A decision must be made about suitability in each case.

Generally, outpatient surgery is best suited for a simple procedure that can be performed within 60 to 90 minutes on a healthy patient who has no other medical problems. In the most uncomplicated situation, the ideal candidate for outpatient surgery is someone who requires only bedrest, food, water and pain medications to become healthy again after an operation.

Why Outpatient Surgery Might Not Be Appropriate Many procedures do not lend themselves to outpatient surgery. Some operations that involve a large abdominal incision, for example, can be performed in 90 minutes, but there is no way you could return home a few hours afterwards.

◆ When surgery cannot be performed on an outpatient basis, it is usually because intensive postoperative monitoring is needed. If you have high blood pressure or heart or lung problems, for example, you need much more careful monitoring after the procedure than could possibly be provided at home.

◆ The magnitude of the procedure may also mean that you will have to receive stronger pain medication than can be given at home.

◆ Some operations pose a greater risk of postoperative complications. In these cases, the procedure should be done in the main operating room, and your surgeon may have to evaluate your condition frequently during the next few days.

Personal Factors If the procedure is one that can be performed on an outpatient basis and risks are not a major concern, other factors must be considered.

◆ *Your age and general physical condition.* In most cases, you should not have any other medical problems.

◆ *Your social and family situation.* If you are being treated as an outpatient, others will have to be willing to help you out at least for the first 24 hours and possibly longer.

◆ *Your attitude toward outpatient surgery.* You have to understand clearly what is expected of you and must be reliable and cooperative. You will have to comply, without fail, with preoperative instructions such as not eating or drinking after midnight the night before the procedure, arriving on time, arranging to have someone drive you home and having someone available to stay with you for the first 24 hours.

YOUR DECISION TO PROCEED

No one is forced to have surgery. Once your surgeon has given you complete information about the proposed procedure and what it will mean to you in the short term and the long term, it is up to you to decide whether you want to go ahead with the operation.

There may be time restrictions—if the surgery involves a biopsy to determine whether you have cancer, time is obviously of the essence—but in most circumstances, you should take all the time you need to reach a decision you are comfortable with. As you make this decision, there are several things you should keep in mind.

Weighing the Risks There are always three main risks to surgery, namely bleeding, infection and death. How high these risks are depends on the nature of the surgery being done.

◆ *Bleeding.* Whenever a surgeon cuts into the skin, some bleeding occurs. Whether there is a risk of *serious* bleeding depends on the area being treated. When a surgeon is operating directly on blood vessels, the chances of bleeding are obviously higher.

Most people do not suffer from any effects of blood loss. Most people can lose 1 pint (500 mL) of blood without adverse effects, and some can lose even more. But any loss of more than 2 pints (1 L) could be serious enough to require a transfusion.

What is of concern to a surgeon is *unexpected* bleeding. In a gallbladder operation, for example, heavy bleeding is not expected, but if a vessel is cut, as much as a pint of blood could be lost. But the risk of unexpected bleeding—which again may not have any bad effect—is perhaps 1 in 500.

◆ *Infection*. Since the skin is the normal barrier that keeps out bacteria, whenever the skin is cut there is some risk that bacteria could get into the body and cause an infection. The infection might affect the incision itself or deeper tissues, particularly in the abdomen.

The risk of infection is no more than 1 or 2 percent. With careful monitoring at home, any infection that does develop can be identified quickly and treated with antibiotics.

◆ *Death*. Even for a healthy person with no other medical problems, there is always a risk of some complication developing during surgery that could lead to death. A blood clot could be released from somewhere in the body, air could get into a blood vessel or there could be an unexpected reaction to a drug. Such things do happen, but the risk is tiny, probably in the range of one occurrence in 10,000 operations.

FACING COMMON FEARS

The normal risks of surgery may be straightforward and few, but when faced with the prospect of "going under the knife," most people have other anxieties. These are perfectly normal, and if you have any of these fears you should feel free to discuss them with your surgeon.

The Unknown Most people don't know exactly where their gallbladder is, let alone what it does except make stones. This can create a great deal of concern when a surgeon explains that the gallbladder has to be removed. Many people wonder, "How am I going to live without a gallbladder?" The fact is, people do very well without a gallbladder.

With clear explanations and perhaps some visual aids, your surgeon should be able to put your mind at ease.

Pain In most types of surgery, the patient will not feel any pain during the procedure. After the operation, the pain is usually due to the incision or the area where the skin was cut. Most of the internal work doesn't arouse sensations of pain.

Pain can be controlled by anesthesia in the operating room and by medications during the recovery period. An infiltration anesthetic may be injected just before you wake up so that you don't feel any stabbing pain at the incision site. Such anesthetics last from 12 to 24 hours, the period when pain is at its worst. Prescription drugs can alleviate pain over the following days.

Something Will Go Wrong Despite all the advances of modern medicine, there is still some danger involved in surgery. There are many stories in the popular press about disasters happening during operations, and these stories generate a lot of anxiety. A man having surgery to one leg went so far as to write with a black magic marker all over the other leg, "Other side. Other side. Other side." Such mishaps are extremely rare.

Something Unexpected Will Be Found This is a secret fear of many patients. With abdominal surgery, for example, many people are afraid the surgeon will find evidence of cancer somewhere. This does happen, but very rarely. A busy surgeon working in a busy surgery unit in a major city may find something unexpected perhaps once or twice a year.

Contaminated Blood Almost all patients wonder whether they will need blood during an operation and whether they can trust the supply to be free of the human immunodeficiency virus (HIV) or other dangerous contaminants. This is a major worry despite the fact that transfusions are almost never needed in outpatient surgery and even though the blood supply is now very well screened.

The risk of hepatitis is greater than the risk of HIV, but the AIDS blood scare of the 1980s changed the way everyone looked at transfusions. One way doctors responded was by being much more conservative about giving blood.

It used to be that if a person's hematocrit (a measure of red blood cells) fell below 30 percent—normal being around 45 in a man and 40 in a woman—a transfusion would be in order. In the past few years, the threshold level has been dropped to 25 percent in adults and even lower with younger patients. To the surprise of many physicians, their patients did just fine with such low levels of red blood cells. Their wounds healed well and they were able to be reasonably active, although they sometimes tired easily.

Disfigurement Any major cut in the skin will leave a scar, but surgical techniques have developed to the point where some procedures leave either no visible scar at all or a scar that is barely noticeable. Most lumps in the breast, for example, can be removed without leaving a major cosmetic deformity.

There may be some disfigurement in cases where the surgeon has to remove a body part or a large piece of tissue, but this has to be balanced against the benefits of the procedure. If the opera-

tion is being performed because of the possibility of cancer, the main concern is clearly whether the cancer can be removed and the patient cured.

TALKING ABOUT ANESTHESIA

One other common fear has to do with anesthesia. There is no shortage of stories in the popular press about horrible reactions or something else going wrong while under anesthesia. Such things do happen but, again, very rarely.

Expressing Your Concerns For both you and your surgeon, explaining what is involved with anesthesia is an important part of the preoperative discussion. If you have concerns at this meeting or afterwards, be open about them. Ask the members of the medical team for as much information as you need to feel comfortable.

Your surgeon will generally have the first conversation with you about the choice of anesthetic. An anesthesiologist will speak to you closer to the day of surgery. Many anesthesiologists go out of their way to meet with patients well in advance and spend quite a bit of time explaining the pros and cons of particular methods.

Personal Preference Some procedures demand a particular method of anesthesia, but in many cases personal preferences can be accommodated.

Some people don't like the thought of losing consciousness and not being able to control their senses. Others are afraid of going to sleep because they are afraid they won't wake up. They'll ask for alternative anesthesia even if general anesthesia would be best.

Some people prefer general anesthesia. One patient, told that her operation could be performed without any discomfort with a local anesthetic that would last 12 to 24 hours, insisted on being completely knocked out. She didn't want to hear requests for instruments, comments on the procedure or anything else going on in the operating room. Another patient also didn't want to hear any talk in the OR. He asked whether he could listen to music on his personal radio. He kept the headphones on throughout the operation, and everything went very smoothly.

In fact, if a local anesthesia is being used, the operating room tends to be quieter than usual, without discussion about extraneous things—the latest movies, politics or the doings of the San Francisco 49ers—common in operations using general anesthesia. Many surgeons make sure there is music playing in the operating room if the procedure involves a local anesthetic.

Selecting an Anesthesiologist The choice of who will give you the anesthetic can vary. In smaller centers, there may not be any choice, either for you as a patient or for the surgeon. Hospitals and surgery centers have various procedures. An anesthesiologist may be assigned according to a rotation system, in which the surgeon has to take the next one available. In other centers, the choice is up to the surgeon.

In most cases, the surgeon can ask for a particular anesthesiologist. When performing hernia surgery, for example, a surgeon might well want to use an anesthesiologist who is comfortable giving epidurals. With this form of anesthesia, the patient is awake and the surgeon can ask him or her to bear down so the surgeon can see where the hernia is and evaluate the repair once it is fixed. Epidurals require particular skills and may take a bit longer to have an effect, so a few anesthesiologists tend to avoid them. When presenting the choices to patients, such anesthesiologists may

subtly push the patients toward general anesthesia.

COMMUNICATING WITH YOUR SURGEON

Some doctors are better communicators than others. Many will try to respond to all kinds of concerns and queries that their patients don't even ask. But in some cases, you may be given only the most basic information if you don't ask.

Some patients are afraid to ask questions because they don't want to appear ill informed or stupid. Some will go so far as to tell their surgeon that they understand everything being said even when it is obvious by their next question that they don't. It is important that you establish a good rapport with your surgeon and that you do not shrink from asking about even the most basic concerns.

It is true that surgeons are sometimes surprised to discover how little people know about how their bodies work, even highly educated people. But they also realize that the American education system delivers very little information about anatomy, health and medicine.

The key is to not be intimidated.

How Much Information Do You Need? Patients vary considerably in their approach to information. Some want to hear about alternative or experimental treatments or procedures that were performed long ago. Others say, "Spare me the details. I'm not interested in the blood and guts. Just do what you have to do and do a good job."

But as a patient, you should have a good understanding of what is going to happen to you so you can understand what to expect afterwards.

What is important is that you consider the full spectrum of what you are undergoing, rather than concentrating on one aspect of the surgery. One patient set to have a hernia repair shortly before Christmas asked all kinds of technical questions, right down to what type of stitches would be used, but little about possible limitations. The day before the surgery, he announced that he had unrefundable plane tickets to visit relatives on the other side of the continent to spend the holidays and recuperate with them. The surgeon informed him that sitting in a plane for a long time, subject to holiday flight delays and other inconveniences, was ill advised two days after surgery, the period when a surgeon is most concerned about complications. As it happened, the patient took the flight, developed normal postoperative swelling, became very concerned, raced to a local hospital and spent hours waiting in the emergency room, only to learn that everything was fine.

Asking the Right Questions When faced with surgery, almost everyone asks if they will have to go to sleep for the operation, where and how big their scar is going to be and whether a blood transfusion might be needed. Most also ask how long the surgery is going to take, even though that doesn't matter much.

Surprisingly, many people do not ask questions about their surgeons, such as where they trained or what their expertise is in doing a particular procedure.

◆ You should make a point of asking whether the surgeon is Board-eligible or Board-certified, because in some states a surgeon can work in a hospital without such qualifications. Lack of Board certification should raise serious concerns about the surgeon's capabilities.

◆ It is worthwhile to ask if within the last couple of years the surgeon has performed the operation you are having.

◆ If you are having a laparoscopic procedure, question your surgeon carefully about what his or her experience has been with these advanced techniques. There are weekend courses where physicians spend 16 hours performing laparoscopic procedures on pigs. Regrettably, a few physicians have taken these courses, then returned home to work on a patient without any help or supervision. This is asking for trouble.

◆ The other areas that should be covered in detail are preparation, the procedure and postoperative care. The last area is particularly important. Always ask what changes are normal after an operation and what would be considered abnormal. If something unusual or untoward should happen at home, you will know to call your surgeon sooner rather than later.

QUESTIONS TO ASK YOUR SURGEON: A CHECKLIST

The Surgeon
◆ Are you Board-certified?
◆ How many cases such as this have you done and what has the success rate been?
◆ How are the other people who will be involved in my care being selected?
◆ Who will be assisting at the surgery?
◆ Who will be giving me the anesthetic and what are her or his qualifications?

Before the Operation
◆ What tests will I need to have before surgery and where do I have them done?
◆ Is there a possibility that my surgery could be delayed or postponed because of emergencies?
◆ Should I take my normal medications before surgery?
◆ Will I need any special equipment at

home after surgery? If so, what, and where can it be obtained?

◆ How long before surgery should I not eat or drink?

The Procedure

◆ What are the potential problems with this type of surgery? In other words, what can go wrong and what can be done to prevent it?

◆ What is the chance of unexpected bleeding?

◆ What type of anesthetic would be best for this procedure?

◆ Where will the incision be and how big a scar will I have?

◆ Will there be drains, stitches or staples that will have to be removed later?

After Surgery

◆ What if I have to be admitted to the hospital?

◆ What can I expect during the first 24 hours and the first week, month and year after surgery?

◆ What is considered normal and what symptoms should I be concerned about?

◆ Who should be called if I have a question or a problem?

◆ How can I reach you in an emergency?

◆ When can I remove my bandage and shower or bathe?

◆ What should I do if my bandage becomes soiled or wet?

◆ How long will I have to be away from work?

◆ How will my life change after surgery?

◆ Will I have to restrict my activities? For how long?

◆ When should I make an appointment to see you in your office after the operation?

3
AT THE SURGERY CENTER

Rosaire F. Macho, RN, and Lynne Macho, RN

What you experience as an outpatient will vary according to the operation you need and according to where your surgery is performed. But for the most part, the process is similar whether you go to a hospital outpatient department or a specialized surgery facility.

TYPES OF OUTPATIENT SURGERY CENTERS

Outpatient surgery is performed in two types of facilities.

Free-Standing Facilities Some surgery centers are truly "free-standing," being entirely separate from any hospital. An advantage of this type of unit is that everything is specifically designed for taking care of outpatients. This eliminates some of the inefficiencies of hospitals, which are designed for taking care of inpatients. These centers are fully equipped to handle emergencies.

Another advantage is that these facilities can become "centers of excellence." Rather than having three or four institutions in an urban area performing orthopedic or breast surgery, for example, one center with a concentration of expertise and experience is efficient and cost effective.

Hospital Outpatient Units Most hospitals have an outpatient surgery center. These outpatient centers often share many of the services available to the rest of the hospital.

One disadvantage of outpatient units that share operating rooms with the hospital's regular surgery department is that emergencies can delay or cancel elective surgery. One other small disadvantage is that when facilities and staff are shared, x-rays or lab tests are sometimes slow to arrive.

The trend today is to separate the outpatient surgical centers more and more from other parts of the hospital. Newer hospital outpatient centers have their own operating rooms, their own radiology services and their own lab testing facilities.

PLANNING FOR YOUR OPERATION

Sometime before the day of your surgery, you will meet with your surgeon in his or her office to discuss and make plans for your operation. Your surgeon should thoroughly describe the procedure you are to have and talk about any complications that might result.

If you have any questions at all about the procedure, now is the time to ask them. Don't wait until the day of the operation to clear up a few concerns that you may have. You may, however, feel so overwhelmed with information at this meeting that you can't even remember the questions you wanted to ask or think of any new ones. If you think of questions later, write them down, get in touch with your surgeon and ask them. It is far better to have everything clear ahead of time.

There also will be a lot of other material to cover at this meeting.

Preoperative Tests Your surgeon will discuss with you whether any tests have to be done. These are usually performed on an outpatient basis before the day of your surgery. Your surgeon's office staff will usually tell you where to have the tests done, which may be at the hospital where you will have your surgery or at an independent laboratory.

These tests may include:
◆ blood work to determine blood counts and chemistries;
◆ an electrocardiogram (EKG) to provide basic information about how your heart is functioning;
◆ a chest x-ray to check the functioning of your lungs, or x-rays of the site of the surgery; and
◆ an analysis of your urine.

If you recently completed any of these tests with another doctor, ask your surgeon whether the tests have to be repeated; a copy of the earlier results may be sufficient.

What to Do about Medications If you are taking medications for a heart condition, insulin for diabetes, steroids or any other medications for some condition unrelated to your surgery, ask your surgeon whether any should be discontinued before your surgery. Also check if there are medications you might need to take with a sip of water the morning of surgery (*see* "Eating and Drinking Before Surgery" below). Make sure your surgeon is aware of all the medications you are currently taking, and do not discontinue any of your medications without consulting your doctor first.

Special Equipment Your surgeon will discuss whether you will need any special equipment after surgery, such as a wheelchair, crutches or a walker. If so, you can make arrangements to have them ready for you ahead of time. If your surgeon thinks it appropriate, you may want to bring them with you on the day of your surgery.

Your surgeon will tell you what other medical supplies you may require for your home recovery period. If dressings or special surgical tape are needed, the hospital or surgical center will generally provide a one- or two-day supply upon discharge. For more supplies, local drugstores usually carry anything you might need.

Eating and Drinking Before Surgery There will be a period before your surgery when you will not be able to eat or drink anything, including water. Usually this period starts at midnight on the night before the operation or at least eight hours before surgery. Check with your surgeon about the specific time for you since it may depend upon the time that your surgery is scheduled.

The reason for going without food and drink is to prevent vomiting during surgery. If you throw up while anesthetized, the stomach contents could enter your lungs. At the very least, this could cause severe respiratory complications during and after the operation.

Pre-Registration Certain surgery centers will ask that you come in a day or more ahead of time to pre-register and fill out any insurance or hospital authorization forms. Bring with you insurance cards and any pre-authorization forms that may be required.

When you come to register, it is sometimes possible to have someone show you the surgery center to help familiarize you with what you'll be going through. Check ahead of time to see if this is possible in your facility.

Making Arrangements for the Day of Surgery After meeting with your surgeon, there are certain arrangements you will want to take care of before your surgery. The most important is to arrange to have a responsible adult accompany you to the surgery center, drive you home and remain with you for the first 24 hours.

You may feel just fine after surgery and think you can make it home on your own. But even if your surgery is being done under a local anesthetic, chances are you will also be receiving some medication to relax you. After receiving sedation, legally you are not allowed to drive.

In many centers, it is also not enough to arrive by yourself and tell the center staff that someone will pick you up later. Your surgery may be canceled if you do.

Getting Yourself Physically Prepared Both surgery and the recovery period proceed much more smoothly if you are in shape. If possible, a few weeks before your operation you should:
◆ For some surgeries, lose weight if you are overweight. This is especially helpful if you are going to have a hernia operation.
◆ Exercise, even if it's only taking long walks. Exercise will improve your circulatory and respiratory systems.
◆ If you smoke, try to stop or reduce your smoking as much as possible.

THE DAY OF SURGERY

Be well prepared before you leave home for the surgery center. Know what you are going to take and who will go with you. Leave lots of time so that you're not rushed.

What to Wear Wear loose, comfortable clothes to the surgery center. Think about where your incisions and dressings will be before choosing what to wear. Comfort and practicality are the key words to keep in mind. You will want to wear only the bare essentials.
◆ Tight underwear, pantyhose, girdles, high heels or any other kind of constricting clothing should be left at home.
◆ If you are having knee, abdominal or hernia surgery, don't wear tight pants. A baggy zipper-down jogging suit is appropriate. In fact, a jogging suit works well for most operations.
◆ Shorts are great for knee surgery, if the weather permits.
◆ If your arm will be in a cast, a shirt with large armholes is best.
◆ Women having laparoscopy may prefer a loose, beltless dress.
◆ Shoes with Velcro fasteners are helpful for patients having arm or hand surgery.

What to Leave at Home You may want to bring make-up with you to the surgery center for the trip home. But the medical team will want to see your natural coloring, so do not apply make-up, nail polish or lipstick on the morning of your operation.
◆ If you wear contact lenses, either remove them at home and wear your eyeglasses or bring your contact lens case and solution with you. You will not be permitted to wear contacts in the operating room.
◆ You will probably be allowed to wear your wedding ring or a Medi-alert bracelet secured with tape into the operating room, but all other jewelry will have to be removed.
◆ It is best to leave valuables at home. Staff at the surgery center will not be able to keep an eye on your valuables or be responsible for them. If you want to

wear a watch, be sure it is an inexpensive one.

◆ If you wear dentures that can be removed, you may choose to leave them at home. You will have to remove them for surgery anyway, since they pose the hazard of slipping back into your throat and blocking your airway when you are asleep.

◆ If you feel you do not want to be seen without your dentures, have the friend or family member who accompanies you keep them for you until after the operation.

Giving the Nurse Your Medical History When you are admitted to the surgery center, a nurse will complete a Nursing Admission Form. This form includes questions about your medical and surgical history, any drug allergies you have and which prescription and non-prescription medications you are taking or have recently taken.

Some of these questions may seem redundant. You will have already gone over your history with your doctor and you may feel that she or he has all that information. The nurses, however, will be taking care of you before and after your surgery, and they also need to know your medical history. They will then be better able to make decisions about planning and delivering safe care. It is better to be doubly sure rather than miss an important fact.

◆ Bring with you a list of the medications you are taking. Write down all the dosages and how often you take the medication.

◆ Also list any medications you are allergic to and the type of reaction you had to each. No one has taken every medication available, so it stands to reason that you can say only which medications you have taken that have caused an adverse reaction. But even if penicillin gave you a rash as a child many years ago, it is important to mention it. Carry a list of

which medications you are allergic to in your wallet or purse at all times.

◆ The nurse will ask you when you last ate or had something to drink. Be honest. Eating or drinking too close to the time of surgery can cause serious complications. If you just couldn't make it through the required waiting period without food, the worst that can happen is that your surgery will be delayed until it is safe to operate.

Completing the Paperwork There will be a number of papers to sign before surgery, and it is important that you understand what you are signing.

◆ One document is the Surgical Consent Form. Read this carefully and make sure you understand exactly what procedure you are having. Of course, your surgeon should have explained what he or she is going to do ahead of time, but the form may contain some unfamiliar medical terminology. If it does, ask to have the terms explained.

Sign the consent form only after you feel comfortable that what it describes is, in fact, the procedure you and your surgeon have discussed. If there is any doubt in your mind, ask to speak to your surgeon.

◆ Every surgical unit has slightly different paperwork. Just remember the rule that each paper has to be read carefully and that you will sign it only after you are sure you understand what it means.

Getting Ready for Surgery After you have finished all your paperwork and your nursing history, your nurse will show you to a room where you will change into a hospital gown and slippers.

◆ Your clothes will be placed in a locker or compartment.

◆ You will be asked to empty your bladder at this time and remove any contact lenses, jewelry and dentures.

◆ A baseline set of vital signs will be

taken, which will include your temperature, pulse rate, respiratory rate and blood pressure.

◆ An anesthesiologist will have discussed the type of anesthesia that will be used and any possible risks or side effects (*see* Chapter 5). Ask as many questions as you need to feel comfortable. Tell her or him any concerns you may have, including any unpleasant experiences you or members of your family may have had with anesthesia, such as persistent nausea or unexplained fevers during or after surgery.

◆ The friend or family member who accompanied you will be shown to the waiting room. Your surgeon will speak with them there after surgery and let them know how everything went.

◆ You will be put on a gurney (a stretcher with wheels) and moved to a preoperative holding area until it is your turn to be taken to the operating room. The holding area may simply be a hospital corridor, so don't be surprised to see many doctors, nurses and other patients in the area.

◆ At some point an intravenous (IV) solution will be started in your arm. This is to provide you with fluids and any medications needed during surgery. The IV will also be used during your recovery period if you should need any medication.

As soon as all these preparations are complete, you will be wheeled into the operating room.

THE OPERATING ROOM

In the operating room, or OR, the surgical team will make sure that everything proceeds smoothly.

Your surgeon will head the team, which may include another doctor serving as a surgical assistant. The anesthesiologist will help position you properly, as well as deliver the anesthetic. The scrub nurse will set up all the instruments the surgeon prefers for the procedure and will generally assist the surgeon during the operation. A circulating nurse will provide whatever supplies are needed and make sure sterile procedures are followed.

◆ Patches attached to wires will be placed on your chest. These connect you to a cardiac monitor to assess your heart rhythm during surgery. A blood pressure cuff will be placed on your arm and a body temperature monitor will be attached to your skin.

◆ If you are having a general anesthetic, the anesthesiologist will put medication in your IV that will make you feel very drowsy. You may be asked to count backwards from 100 until you are asleep. Once you are asleep, the nurses and operating room technicians will position you in the correct and safe position.

◆ Your surgical site will be washed with a surgical disinfectant. For some operations, some portion of skin may be shaved to reduce the possibility of bacteria entering your surgical wound. (When you see your surgical site afterwards, you may see the remains of the surgical scrub and newly shaved skin. Some scrubs will make the area around your incision appear a yellowish brown. It washes off easily.)

THE RECOVERY ROOM

When your surgery is complete, you will be taken to the Post-Anesthesia Care Unit, more commonly known as the recovery room. The nurses here will monitor your condition closely, frequently checking your vital signs—your blood pressure, temperature, pulse and respiration.

◆ You may have an oxygen mask, an EKG monitor and an oxygen monitor on, and your IV will still be infusing.

◆ After about a half-hour to an hour, depending on the anesthetic used, you will gradually wake up. You will feel quite sleepy, but this should pass fairly quickly. You may also feel cold, since the operating room is kept cool. The nurses will give you more warm blankets if you need them or if your temperature is low.

◆ If you are feeling pain or nausea, let your nurse know so that she or he can take measures to alleviate your discomfort.

◆ The head of your bed will be gradually raised (depending on your type of surgery) and you will be asked to take frequent deep breaths to help keep your lungs clear.

◆ You may be offered ice chips or water to drink to find out how well you tolerate fluids. It's best to start slowly even if you are thirsty and do not feel nauseated.

When you are wide enough awake and your vital signs are stable, the recovery room nurses will transfer you to the Same-Day Surgery Unit, where you will be taken care of until you are ready to be discharged.

THE SAME-DAY SURGERY UNIT

When you are sufficiently alert, you will be asked to sit up with your feet over the side of the bed. If you are not too dizzy, you may be asked to take a few steps to see how steady you are on your feet.

It is normal to feel a little woozy when you first get up, but you should be able to walk a short distance, depending on your type of surgery and your physical condition before surgery.

Depending on the kind of institution you are in, you will usually be placed in a recliner or a simplified bed. The family member or friend who accompanied you can join you at this point.

Making Sure You Are Stable The nurses will continue to check your vital signs at regular intervals to assess your recovery from the anesthesia. They will also check your dressing to make sure that it is dry and in place.

◆ Depending on the type of surgery you had, the type of anesthetic and the protocol of the institution you are in, you may be assisted to the bathroom and asked to urinate before you are discharged.

◆ If at any time you feel that your bladder is full but you can't pass urine, be sure to let your nurse know so he or she can take appropriate measures. These may include something as simple as having the water running in the bathroom or possibly passing a urinary catheter into your bladder. You may think that you couldn't possibly have any urine because you haven't had anything to drink for hours, but you probably received several quarts (litres) of fluid through your IV in both the operating room and the recovery room.

Managing Pain and Nausea You may experience pain and/or nausea after surgery. Be sure to keep the nurses informed of this so they can properly assess your pain and nausea and take appropriate actions to keep you comfortable.

◆ They have orders from your surgeon to administer medications as needed. If the pain medication isn't working, they may get in contact with your surgeon to change to a more effective medication.

◆ In rare instances, the amount of pain or nausea you have may mean that you have to stay at the hospital a little longer than expected or even be admitted to stay overnight. Your nurse will assess your condition and make the appropriate arrangements with your surgeon and the admitting staff.

Discharge When you are sufficiently recovered from anesthesia and are ready to be discharged, your IV will be removed and your nurse will review your discharge instructions.

She or he will instruct you on:

◆ what medications your doctor has prescribed;

◆ when you can remove your bandage and bath or shower;

◆ how to apply a fresh dressing if needed;

◆ how to use any special equipment your doctor may have ordered;

◆ what symptoms or complications you should be aware of; and

◆ who to contact in case of an emergency.

If there are any instructions you don't understand, be sure to ask the nurse. It is better to have your questions answered before you leave the surgery unit than to wait until you get home.

The nurse will also tell you when you are to see the surgeon in the office. *Be sure to keep your follow-up appointments.* They are very important to the success of your surgery.

COMMON CONCERNS AFTER SURGERY

A major concern of many patients and their families is how they will know if something is abnormal. Surgeons and nurses are frequently asked, "How much bleeding is too much? How will I know if the wound is infected? What if my pain is too much for me to manage? How much can I do when I get home?"

Most patients do just fine at home and have minimal complications or no complications at all. Most people are more comfortable in their own homes than in a hospital and recover nicely. Knowing what to watch for will decrease many of the concerns you may have.

Mild Nausea This is the most common complaint after surgery.

◆ To help avoid or minimize nausea, resume drinking and eating slowly. Start with small sips of clear liquids. If

you can tolerate that, move on to soft and bland foods such as crackers, noodles, rice or jelly for the first 24 hours.

◆ Nausea becomes a concern if you vomit frequently or for a prolonged period and cannot keep liquids down. If this happens, try resting your stomach for 30 minutes or an hour. Then try sips of clear liquids again.

◆ If the vomiting continues and you can't even tolerate water, notify your surgeon.

◆ Once the nausea has passed, advance slowly to your normal diet.

◆ Children are at a greater risk for the effects of dehydration. Any continued vomiting should be reported to your surgeon immediately.

Pain Each surgery has its own set of "normals" in regard to pain. How much pain is too much depends on your type of surgery, your pain tolerance, your age and your physical condition. Discuss your situation with the surgeon before your operation so you will have an idea of what to expect once you are home.

◆ It is always a good idea to take the pain medication prescribed for you with food to avoid nausea.

◆ Narcotic pain medications can also be constipating, so ask your surgeon for suggestions on how to offset this problem.

◆ If you find that the prescribed pain relievers are not working, contact your surgeon.

AT HOME

With the wide range of operations being performed on an outpatient basis, there are few hard-and-fast rules to follow once you are at home. Your previous condition and the nature of your surgery will determine what you can and can't do.

◆ Always check with your surgeon for

specific care instructions. Some of these will have been explained by the nurse upon discharge. These might include no heavy lifting if you have had a hernia repair or driving restrictions if you have had eye surgery.

◆ It is not unusual to feel weak and tired when you leave the hospital or surgery center. That is one reason why it is imperative that a responsible adult drive you home and remain with you for the first 24 hours.

◆ During those first 24 hours after receiving anesthesia (or while you are taking narcotic pain medication), you should not drink alcohol, drive or make any important decisions.

◆ Plan on resting for the remainder of the day of surgery.

◆ Do not plan on resuming any of your usual activities for the first few days. Make arrangements to have someone help you.

◆ It is important that you move around a bit when you are at home. Unless otherwise instructed by your surgeon, getting up to go to the bathroom and taking short walks around the room will help promote good circulation.

◆ Taking deep breaths and coughing every couple of hours will help keep your lungs clear.

WHEN TO CALL YOUR SURGEON

You should be able to manage most situations at home, but you should call your surgeon when:

◆ Your wound appears infected. The area around the incision may be red and hot and you may have fever or chills. A foul-smelling or thick green or yellow fluid may also start to drain from the wound.

◆ You experience severe nausea, especially after taking pain medication.

◆ You have any other concerns about your postoperative care.

When There Is an Emergency There are times when you must get in touch with your surgeon immediately. Your discharge instructions will list telephone numbers where your surgeon may be reached. These should include her or his office number and a number to call at night and on weekends.

It is possible that if you call with an emergency during the night or over a weekend, your surgeon may not be available. But another surgeon will be able to tell you what to do.

Emergency Situations Naturally, if you cannot be aroused at all, a family member or friend should make sure you receive immediate medical attention.

Get in touch with your surgeon promptly:

◆ If you start bleeding a great deal. A large amount of bright red blood or clots may appear. If this happens, apply direct pressure to the incision site. If possible, elevate the affected body part while you summon help.

◆ If you have acute, severe pain uncontrolled by the prescribed pain medication.

◆ If the wound opens.

◆ If a limb on which surgery was performed becomes blue or numb.

◆ If you have a fever with a temperature higher than 100.4°F (38°C).

4
PREPARING YOUR CHILD FOR SURGERY

Rosaire F. Macho, RN, *and Lynne Macho,* RN

———◇———

More and more surgical procedures are being performed on children on an outpatient basis. Tonsils and adenoids are removed, hernias are repaired and many other procedures are performed safely without a hospital stay.

The process of going through surgery is much the same for children as it is for adults (*see* Chapter 3). All the paperwork, for example, is a standard procedure no matter what the age of the patient. Other parts of the process are very different, however, because children have children's fears and questions. They are not "little adults."

A well-respected pediatrician, Dr. T. Berry Brazelton, describes the feelings a child has about hospitalization and the unknown in his book *To Listen to a Child*: "The unknown and the unexpected is far more frightening for children than is fear of pain for which they are prepared, even though they may protest more vigorously at the time. In addition to the anxiety which is dispelled by preparation for each step in such an experience, the child's trust in her parents and their ability to protect her are tremendously reinforced if the child has seen that they themselves are not overwhelmed by this strange, new experience."

CHILDREN'S CONCERNS

How children react to surgery depends a lot on their age and developmental characteristics. As children grow older, their fears about surgery change.

The First Three Years These are the most vulnerable years. Children are not always old enough to understand what will be done to them, but they are old enough to remember the experience. Children at this age are most concerned about separation. Separation anxiety is at its height in this age group.
♦ Assure your child often that you will return.
♦ It is helpful for the child to see and handle new and strange equipment whenever possible.
♦ Bring a favorite toy or stuffed animal to the hospital.

Four to Seven In these years, separation is easier for children simply because they understand more. The fear of mutilation and loss of a part of their body is more frightening to a child now. They will need to feel some control over their environment and what is happening to them.
♦ Talk to your child directly about what will happen and involve him or her in decisions.
♦ Allow them to handle new and strange equipment.
♦ Rehearsing what might happen ahead of time will be reassuring. Be direct and matter-of-fact, saying, "The doctor will put a mask on you that will help you to sleep" or "The nurses will take you to the operating room on a red cart and I'll go with you right to the operating room door."
♦ Bring a favorite toy to the hospital.

Eight to Twelve At this age, children are developing and building their self-esteem. They may feel that it is threatened or changed because of having surgery. The child needs to feel some control over the situation.

◆ This may be provided by having a parent nearby and by having all procedures explained to the child's satisfaction.

◆ A hospital orientation is very helpful for this age group, as it allows them to feel that control they need to have over their lives (i.e., they acquire information and have a chance to ask questions). It also serves to defuse the scare stories that are so much a part of a school-aged child's life.

Thirteen to Eighteen Adolescents are very concerned about their body image. They will often minimize the severity of a problem. They also greatly value their independence. They often want more information than their surgeon gives them about what's going to happen.

FACING YOUR OWN FEARS

Surgery on oneself is usually a frightening and threatening experience to deal with. Surgery on one's children holds a whole new set of fears.

While you do your best to calm your child's fears about surgery, it is important for your child to know that you aren't afraid or overwhelmed by the thought of surgery either. You will have to approach the experience openly and truthfully with information that is as unfrightening as possible.

Separation Often, the biggest fear parents have is separation from their child. The most common questions nurses hear from parents in the outpatient surgery unit are "When can I see my child again?" and "Will my child be left alone?"

The feeling that you will be unable to control what happens to your child once she or he is out of your sight is often overwhelming. You worry that no one could provide care as well as you would or give your child the warm personal attention that you would. Allowing the hospital staff and your surgeon and anesthesiologist to take your child away for surgery means that you have to place your trust in them and allow them to act for you in your child's best interests. This is difficult to do.

To help yourself maintain a sense of control in your child's life now, spend as much time together as you can and reassure your child that you are waiting for and always thinking of her or him. To help yourself get through the waiting and deal with the feeling of helplessness, look for and get support from a spouse, another family member or a close friend. It's okay to admit that you're afraid, but you still need to be outwardly strong in front of your child.

Something Will Go Wrong Parents worry about whether their child will come out of the anesthesia safely or that something will go wrong during surgery. Every parent has these fears, and it is difficult to accept that you cannot control the outcome of surgery.

The control you do have in this situation is the power to choose a surgeon and an anesthesiologist with the best qualifications. You need to do a little homework as a parent. The anesthesiologist and the surgeon should both be Board-certified in their specialties. The anesthesiologist should be experienced in performing pediatric anesthesia.

Beyond taking these steps, you must trust the surgeon and the surgical staff to do the best job possible.

How Much Do I Tell My Child? Many parents ask, "Won't I just frighten my child by explaining too much in advance?" The answer is that you should always be honest with your child about new and potentially frightening things.

Often parents don't want to prepare their children because they themselves find it hard to face the coming separation and the surgery and can't bear to discuss it. But the rule of thumb is that a child will do much better when he or she knows what to expect in an experience, especially one that involves painful procedures. They may protest about the pain or the procedure, but at least if things are expected, the child will know that you have been truthful and can be trusted.

LEARNING ABOUT WHAT WILL HAPPEN

Most health care workers realize that education and familiarity with the process will make the surgical experience much less frightening for children and their families. So in most surgery centers, children and parents can receive some preoperative teaching. This makes a scary process much less frightening.

Using Books and Booklets Many surgery centers and pediatric surgery offices offer colorful booklets for parents and children describing what to expect before, during and after surgery. Books about children having surgery are also available from the hospital or your local library or bookstore so that you can go through them with your child at home.

Touring the Surgery Center Some centers allow families to take a tour before the operation, letting the children handle the equipment they will see when they come back for surgery. Some put on puppet shows designed to set young minds at ease. Check ahead of time whether your surgery center offers this service.

Role Playing With younger children, you can prepare for the surgical experience at home by role playing. You might have your child pretend to be the patient while you play the doctor. Children do not always talk easily with a doctor; they are more likely to tell *you* what makes them feel afraid, knowing that you will give them the reassurance they need.

BEFORE SURGERY

Before the day of surgery, you will meet with your child's surgeon to discuss the procedure your child will be undergoing. The discussion should be thorough. Make sure you understand why the operation is being done and all the possible complications.

Ask questions to find out everything you can about what will be done. This will give you the information you need to prepare your child. It is helpful if you've written down questions as you thought of them before the meeting and take the list with you. Be sure to also let your surgeon know of any fears you may have.

History At this meeting, the surgeon will ask you about your child's medical and surgical history so that he or she will have a complete picture of your child's health and any special needs your child may have.

The surgeon will want to know whether your child is taking any medications and how long he or she has been taking them. If your child is on medication, bring a list with the drug names, dosages and information about how often the medication is taken. The surgeon will let you know which medications your child should or should not take on the morning of surgery. To ensure your child's safety, it is very important to be honest and thorough when answering these questions. Your surgeon must have a complete and accurate history.

Special Tests and Equipment The surgeon should also discuss any lab tests that might have to be done before surgery. As with adults, these are usually done on an outpatient basis several days before the operation.

The need for bandages or special equipment may also be covered at the meeting.

AT THE HOSPITAL

You will be asked to report to the surgery center with your child a few hours before the time scheduled for the operation. Most centers try to schedule children's surgery as the first cases of the day because it's hard to explain to hungry young children why they cannot have breakfast. If you are the first case, expect to arrive by about 6:45 a.m.

Fasting Your child will have gone without food or drink since midnight. With infants, the fasting period may be only four to six hours. They are more prone to dehydration and are less able to go without fluids for long periods.

Meeting with the Nurse The nurses will be waiting for you when you arrive and will help you get ready, making sure that all your paperwork and lab work are in order.

The nurses will give you and your child a running commentary of what to expect next. They will take a short nursing history from you, covering your child's health, medications and any allergies. The anesthesiologist will later ask you many of these same questions, and you may begin to feel you have said everything there is to say at least a hundred times. But it is very important to answer all these questions fully. Everyone on the medical team needs

this information. Although nurses do not operate independently, they often have to make decisions about your child's care before and after surgery, and they need your background information to make such decisions safely.

Consenting to Surgery A nurse will give you the surgical consent form to sign. Be sure to read the procedure that is listed and make sure that your child's name is on the form before signing it. If the procedure named or the medical terminology on the form does not sound like what you and your child's doctor have discussed, don't sign. Do not be afraid about making people angry with you.

Ask to have the wording explained to you if it is unclear. If the procedure is still not what you understood it would be, have the nurse get in touch with the surgeon to clear up any discrepancy. Only when you feel clear about what is to be done, sign the consent form.

There may be other forms requiring your signature, and the same rule applies. Sign each only after you have thoroughly read it and understand it.

Talking about Anesthesia The anesthesiologist will ask you questions about your child's health, medications, allergies and previous experience with anesthesia.

The anesthesiologist is an important part of the pediatric surgical team. He or she will be the person you hand your child over to at the operating room door. His or her face will usually be the last face your child sees before going to sleep and may be the first face your child sees when waking up after surgery.

Getting a Shot The nurses will not usually take blood pressure or do anything invasive before surgery, but they will measure your child's pulse and breathing rate. They will also give some preoperative medication. In older children this may be delivered through an intravenous line, but is often given in the form of a shot. Don't tell your child that the shot won't hurt. It will, so be honest. Say something such as "This is going to hurt a little, but it will help to make you sleepy so your surgery won't hurt."

With older children, nurses may give choices about where a shot may be given. This lets the child experience a little autonomy and control. With younger children, it is usually best not to give too many choices, since the choice will often be to not have the shot at all. Parents may be asked to hold younger children while the shots are being given and reassure them and to hug and comfort them afterwards.

Getting Ready Just before surgery, a nurse will ask you to help dress your child in a hospital gown. Many preschoolers and school-age children resist giving up their underpants, so most surgery centers allow them to keep their underpants on until they are under anesthesia.

You will need to remove barrettes, bobby pins and jewelry. The nurse will also ask you about, and may check for, any loose teeth, especially if your child is between six and eight and is losing her or his first teeth. Retainers or orthodontic rubber bands will be removed, since they could be knocked free and cause breathing problems during the operation.

Stay with your child and be reassuring through all these unfamiliar procedures. It often helps for a preschool child to have a special toy or blanket to hold onto for comfort.

Adolescents may ask a lot of questions about everything that is done, and the nurses will usually try to include them in as much of the discussion as possible and to give them choices to help maintain their independence and need for knowledge. Because adolescents may be self-conscious about their bodies, they will probably want privacy when they are changing into the hospital gown. They may not even want a parent around.

Going to the Operating Room Your child will be placed on a stretcher with the side rails up and will be wheeled either briefly to a holding area or directly to the operating room. Children are never left alone. Someone will always be talking with them and reassuring them.

Your child may bring a favorite toy or animal along for comfort, and you may walk alongside the stretcher to the doors of the operating room.

A nurse will show you where the waiting room is. A nurse and the surgeon will come here after the operation to let you know how everything went. A nurse will usually try to contact you as soon as word comes from the operating room so that you can set your mind at ease.

In the Operating Room The anesthesiologist will be waiting in the operating room to put your child to sleep. Anesthesiologists are aware of the fears children have about surgery and will talk with them and make them feel comfortable as they begin to fall asleep.

Once your child is asleep, the anesthesiologist will attach a heart monitor and an oxygen monitor to keep track of heart rhythm, breathing rate and the amount of oxygen in the blood.

The nurses and technicians will then place your child in the correct and safe position for surgery. His or her body will be covered with surgical drapes, with only the area to be operated on left uncovered. Except in the case of ear, nose and throat operations, the operative site will be washed with a surgical scrub to disinfect the skin. You may see traces of this around the incision after surgery. It is nothing to worry about and will wash off.

THE RECOVERY ROOM

Once the surgery is over, the anesthesiologist will begin to waken your child. Your child will then be transferred on a stretcher to the nurses in the recovery room.

It is important to let children know ahead of time that they will be in a different room when they wake up and will see some unfamiliar faces asking questions such as, "What is your name?" Their intravenous (IV) line will still be in place in case the nurses need to give medication. They may also still have an oxygen monitor in place, which may be left on until they're fully awake. Children tend to be frightened by all the wires and tubes, so before they are transferred to the same-day surgery unit the tubes are usually removed.

◆ The nurses will monitor breathing, heart rate and temperature frequently and will stay with your child to make sure she or he won't be frightened. In some centers, parents are permitted to see their children as soon as they awaken.

◆ Your child may be cold or have a slightly lowered temperature because the operating room is kept cool. The nurses will provide warm hospital gowns and blankets.

◆ Your child may experience some pain and nausea upon waking. The nurses will assess both conditions and give the appropriate medications to relieve the symptoms. These will usually be given through the IV, since fluids or medications taken by mouth probably will not yet be tolerated.

THE SAME-DAY SURGERY UNIT

Once your child is sufficiently awake, the monitors will be removed and he or she will be transferred on a stretcher back to the same-day surgery unit and put into a bed with side rails. It is important for you to stay with your child now and reassure him or her that everything is all right. Your child may need a familiar toy or book close at hand.

◆ The nurses will continue to monitor your child's heart rate, breathing and temperature to make sure everything is normal.

◆ The nurses will check the surgical dressing and examine it for signs of bleeding. It is helpful for you to look at it too so you will have a basis for comparison once you get home.

◆ As your child begins to become more alert, the nurses will have him or her start to sit up.

Children are first asked to dangle their feet over the side of the bed. If they don't feel dizzy, they are asked to take a few steps to see how steady they are. It is normal for children to feel a little woozy or wobbly on their feet at this point, but if they've been in good health before surgery, they should be able to take a few steps.

◆ Deep breathing and moving around are very important and should be encouraged. Sitting up and walking help clear the lungs of the effects of anesthesia. Your child may not want to do either of these things because it may make the incision hurt. You, along with the nurses, may have to be imaginative in getting your child's cooperation. You might try to have your child imagine taking the deep breath they would have to take before blowing up a big balloon. The nurses will have other ideas for you and may even have some special devices such as an "incentive spirometer" designed specifically for the job.

Dealing with Pain There is a common perception that children don't feel pain as acutely as adults. This is not true. The nurses in the same-day surgery unit will be assessing your child's pain and will have instructions from the surgeon to give pain medications as needed.

As long as your child isn't vomiting or feeling nauseated, these medications will usually be given by mouth. If nausea or vomiting make that impossible, the nurse may give the medication by an injection or through an IV.

Be sure to let the nurses know when your child is in pain and also whether the pain medications are working.

Dealing with Nausea Children often experience nausea or vomiting after anesthesia, so once your child is sufficiently awake the nurses usually begin to give fluids or ice chips slowly. They will not force your child to eat or drink and will encourage you to take it slow with food and liquids as well.

If Hospital Admission Is Necessary In rare cases, pain or nausea that can't be controlled by the usual measures may mean that your child has to stay in hospital overnight. If this should happen, the nurses will make arrangements with your child's surgeon and the admitting staff. Plan to stay with your child for as long as she or he is hospitalized. Separation is very difficult and traumatic for children, especially after having an operation.

GOING HOME

The nurses will prepare you for discharge as soon as your child has recovered sufficiently from the anesthesia, which means that his or her vital signs are stable, pain is under control and he or she is awake, isn't vomiting and has no fever or nausea.

Discharge A set of discharge instructions will be given to you, similar to the instructions described for adults in Chapter 3. These instructions should cover:

♦ Any medications your child might need, such as painkillers or antibiotics.
♦ When and if to remove any bandages.
♦ What signs or symptoms of complications you should call the surgeon about.
♦ What to look for and who to call in an emergency. The nurse should include both the surgeon's office number and a number to call at night and on weekends.
♦ When your child should see the surgeon for a follow-up appointment.
♦ What activities have to be restricted.

Ask the nurse to clarify any instructions that are not completely clear.

The First Day When you get home, your child will normally feel tired and a little weak and should rest for the remainder of the day. One parent or a responsible adult should plan to be with the child for at least the first 24 hours to watch for any problems. Your child will also need you close by. Younger children may be whiney or clingy for a day or more after surgery.

Your child may still feel a little nauseated at home. This is not a concern unless it is accompanied by an inability to keep any food or fluids down. Be aware that children are at a much greater risk than adults for the effects of dehydration, so *any persistent nausea or vomiting should be reported to your doctor immediately.*

Diet Begin giving your child clear liquids, such as jelly, broth, clear soda or juice. When these are tolerated, move on to soft, easily digested foods such as crackers or toast, and gradually advance to a normal diet.

Pain Your child may have some pain for a few days after surgery, which should be eased by the medications prescribed on discharge. If the medication doesn't work well or doesn't work at all, notify your surgeon.

Getting Back to Normal Talk with the surgeon about when your child may go back to school and get involved in regular activities. Your surgeon will give you a good idea of the time frame to expect, based on your child's age, general health and the nature of the operation.

When to Call the Surgeon As with adults (*see* Chapter 3), you should be able to manage most minor medical situations as they arise at home, but call the surgeon if:

◆ The wound appears infected. The signs include an incision that gets red and feels hot to the touch, a thick green or yellow fluid draining from the wound and fever or chills.
◆ Nausea is severe, especially after taking pain medication.
◆ You have any other concerns about you child's care.

Get in touch with your surgeon *immediately* if:

◆ You can't rouse your child at all.
◆ There is a lot of bleeding. If this happens, apply direct pressure to the incision site. If possible, elevate the affected body part while you call for help.
◆ The wound opens.

◆ The limb on which the surgery was performed becomes blue or numb.
◆ An acute or severe pain can't be controlled by the prescribed medication.
◆ Your child develops a fever with a temperature higher than 100.4°F (38°C).

QUESTIONS TO ASK YOUR PEDIATRIC SURGEON

◆ What tests must my child have before surgery and where will they be done?
◆ Should my child take normal medications before the operation?
◆ How long before surgery should my child not eat or drink?
◆ Will we need any special equipment at home? If so, what, and where can it be obtained?
◆ Will my child's activities have to be restricted after surgery? For how long?
◆ When will it be okay to remove the bandages and have a bath or shower?
◆ What should I do if the bandage gets soiled or wet?
◆ What symptoms should I be concerned about after surgery?
◆ Where can I reach you in an emergency?
◆ When should I bring my child in to see you again?

Brazelton, T. Berry. *To Listen to a Child: Understanding the Normal Problems of Growing Up*. 8th ed. New York: Addison-Wesley, 1984, p. 170.

5
ANESTHESIA

Robert S. Dorian, MD

When people are told they need surgery, the first questions that spring to mind are often about anesthesia. How will I go to sleep? How will I feel when I wake up? Will I feel anything at all with a local anesthetic? What's an epidural? Will anesthesia make me feel nauseated? Is it safe?

The thought of surgery and anesthesia can sometimes be overwhelming. But keep in mind that anesthesia is extremely safe. In the United States, about 25

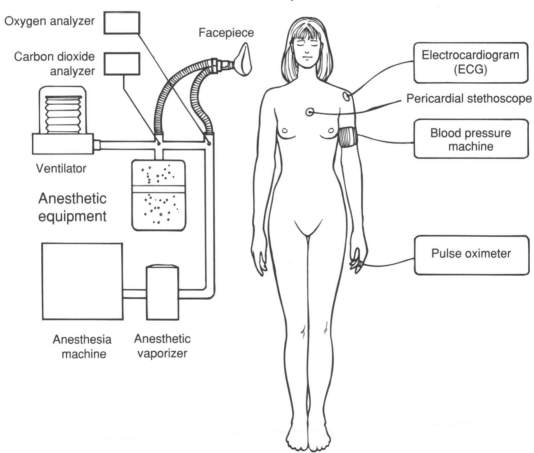

The surgical center, showing typical layout with placement of equipment

million anesthetics are performed on an outpatient basis every year, with a safety record that is nearly perfect. This record is attributable to extensive monitoring of your vital signs with state-of-the-art equipment and to anesthesiologists trained to make informed medical decisions that keep you safe and comfortable during surgery.

The art and science of anesthesia ranks among America's greatest contributions to mankind. It's hard to believe, but only 150 years ago there was no anesthesia at all. Surgery was crude and painful and had to be performed quickly. Soon after the first anesthetic was demonstrated in Boston, the news spread rapidly around the world. Without anesthesia and the professionals who fostered the specialty, surgery could never have advanced and flourished as it has.

TYPES OF ANESTHESIA

Anesthesia means loss of sensation. Part or all of your body can be made completely insensible to pain, for as long or as short a time as necessary, by using various medications to block the conduction of pain and feeling through nerve pathways from the body to the brain. They may also provide amnesia about the actual procedure.

There are three main types of anesthesia.

Local Anesthesia This is used for minor surgery on or near the skin, such as removing a mole or small lump. The anesthesia is achieved by injecting a drug directly into the tissue to numb only the local area.

With local anesthesia you are awake throughout the surgical procedure. If the operation is extensive or if you feel anxious, you may choose to have intravenous sedation along with the local anesthesia. This means that your anes-

thesiologist will deliver mild sedatives directly into the bloodstream to help you relax. You may even doze during the procedure.

One of the advantages of local anesthesia is that very little medication is required, so recovery is immediate and side effects are minimal.

Regional Anesthesia This refers to the use of anesthetics to numb a group of nerves that control an entire region of your body, such as an arm or, quite frequently, both legs from the waist down.

There are two main types of regional anesthesia, spinal and epidural. Both types work by injecting local anesthetic near the nerves coming from the spinal cord. With both types you will be numb from the waist down. This is ideal for surgery involving the lower half of the body, such as the repair of an inguinal hernia, urological procedures or for knee arthroscopy.

Spinal anesthesia is given as a single injection, whereas epidural anesthesia has the advantage of being administered continuously through a tiny flexible tube, or catheter, placed into your epidural space through the skin of your lower back. The timing of the anesthesia can then be tailored to the exact requirements of the surgery.

Regional anesthesia does not put you to sleep. As with a local anesthetic, however, your anesthesiologist can make you as drowsy as you wish by injecting medications intravenously. Having regional anesthesia does not necessarily mean that you will be aware of anything that goes on in the operating room.

Both types of regional anesthesia are extremely safe. Contrary to popular belief, it is not possible to become paralyzed from spinal or epidural anesthesia. It is possible to get a temporary headache from either one of them, but even this is unlikely. Neither anesthetic

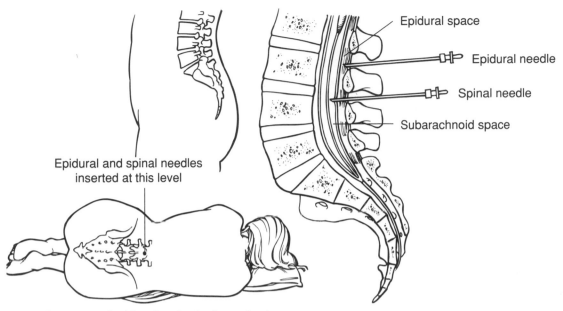

Epidural space

Epidural needle

Spinal needle

Subarachnoid space

Epidural and spinal needles inserted at this level

Placement of epidural and spinal anesthesia

will cause any back pain or injury. In fact, epidural anesthesia is sometimes used to relieve chronic back pain. After regional anesthesia, the skin on your back will be no more tender than the skin on your arm would be after a blood test.

Regional anesthesia wears off slowly, which gives you pain relief immediately after the operation. In about an hour or two, the numbness and sedation are completely worn off and you will be ready for discharge from the recovery room.

Regional anesthesia with intravenous sedation is one of the most pleasant ways to undergo surgery. It is the method most anesthesiologists choose for themselves when they have surgery in the lower half of the body.

General Anesthesia This is what most people think of when they hear that someone is "under anesthesia." General anesthesia means that in addition to not feeling any pain, you are unconscious. Your body and brain are deeply asleep.

You cannot see, feel or hear anything that goes on in the operating room. You do not even dream while under general anesthesia.

General anesthesia can be administered in two ways. Liquid medication may be injected into a vein, or the vapors of an anesthetic gas mixed with oxygen may be breathed through a mask.

General anesthesia is the most frequent type performed in the United States today. It is safe for people of all ages, from newborns to the elderly. General anesthesia for outpatient surgery uses short-acting medications that wear off quickly and have minimal side effects, which means that you recover rapidly and can be sent home as soon as possible after your operation.

THE ROLE OF THE ANESTHESIOLOGIST

To better understand what goes on in the operating room, it helps to distinguish between an anesthetist and an anesthesiologist. An anesthetist is any person who administers the anesthesia. This person might be an anesthesiologist or a certified registered nurse anesthetist (CRNA).

Certified Registered Nurse Anesthetist
A CRNA has a minimum of a bachelor's degree in science. Eighty-five percent of all current programs are master's degree programs leading to a certification exam. There are also continuing education and recertification requirements.

A CRNA is usually an employee of the hospital, but he or she may be an employee of a physicians' group whose activities are focused mainly in the operating room. CRNAs perform their duties only under the direct supervision of a medical doctor, usually the surgeon or an anesthesiologist.

CRNAs are highly qualified to administer anesthesia and do so competently and safely. Half of all anesthetics given every year, and 85 percent of all anesthetics in rural areas, are given by CRNAs.

The Anesthesiologist An anesthesiologist is a medical doctor who has specialized in the field of anesthesiology. An anesthesiologist has many medical responsibilities, one of which is the administration of anesthesia in the operating room.

An anesthesiologist's training is extensive. After medical school there is one year of clinical training, or internship, in either medicine or surgery, then three years of residency training in anesthesia. Many anesthesiologists choose to train for an additional one or two years in a subspecialty such as pediatric or obstetrical anesthesia. After passing rigorous written and oral examinations, the anesthesiologist is certified by the American Board of Anesthesiology.

The greater depth of training of the anesthesiologist allows her or him to perform duties out of the operating room, such as pre- and postoperative care or the management of an intensive care unit.

In the Operating Room The anesthesiologist is not simply the person who puts you to sleep. He or she is the doctor who takes care of you in the operating room. While the surgeon focuses on the technical aspects of your operation, the anesthesiologist focuses on you.

It is your anesthesiologist who guides you through surgery and brings you back safely and reliably to consciousness. The anesthesiologist manages your vital signs and, if necessary, administers blood transfusions.

There are few times in your life when you will be watched so closely or monitored so carefully as when you are under the care of an anesthesiologist. He or she is constantly vigilant and can immediately diagnose and treat any medical situations that may arise during surgery.

Monitoring Your Vital Signs The most important vital signs monitored in the operating room are blood pressure, heart rate, respiration and temperature. Current technology allows us to monitor these vital signs non-invasively, that is, without entering the body or piercing the skin. Microchip-controlled devices are so accurate and sensitive that even the slightest variation in an array of body functions can be detected instantly.
♦ *Blood Pressure.* This is monitored with a pneumatic blood pressure cuff placed around your arm or leg. It automatically inflates every two to five minutes for a continuous and precise record of your blood pressure throughout the operation.
♦ *Heart Rate.* This is monitored with a continuous electrocardiogram (EKG). Three small wires are attached to your

skin with sticky pads. These wires lead to a cardiac monitor that displays your heart rate and rhythm. The shape of the electrocardiogram tracing provides information about the state of the heart muscle and about the blood flow through the coronary arteries.

◆ *Breathing.* Two devices measure lung function.

The pulse oximeter is a device that fits on your fingertip. It reads the amount of oxygen in the bloodstream instantly and continuously.

The end-tidal carbon dioxide monitor measures the amount of carbon dioxide in your exhaled breath and gives an accurate picture of your metabolic level.

These two non-invasive monitors have revolutionized anesthesia and have raised safety to new heights. They are indispensable and are now required by law in all operating rooms.

◆ *Temperature.* The anesthesiologist will maintain your body temperature at a constant level by using sensitive temperature probes and controlling the heat in the operating room. This will help you wake up comfortably at a normal body temperature.

MEETING WITH YOUR ANESTHESIOLOGIST

You will have the opportunity to meet with your anesthesiologist in person either a few days before the surgery, when you have your pre-admission testing, or on the day of surgery. There are several areas to cover at this important preoperative interview.

◆ *Medical background.* It is at this meeting that the anesthesiologist will evaluate your general medical health, the condition for which you are receiving surgery and any chronic medical problems you may have such as asthma, diabetes or high blood pressure.

◆ *Types of anesthesia.* You will have the chance to ask questions about the risks and benefits of the different types of anesthesia and discuss which one is most appropriate for you. The choice of local, regional or general anesthesia for your particular operation depends on many factors, including the part of your body being operated on and how long the operation will take.

◆ *Costs.* Anesthesiologists are physician specialists, just like cardiologists or pediatricians, and most are self-employed professionals rather than hospital employees. So you will probably be sent a bill separate from that of your surgeon. The anesthesiologist will be glad to discuss fees with you and can help you process any insurance papers.

THE DAY OF SURGERY

If you haven't had a previous appointment, you will meet your anesthesiologist at the surgical center to discuss your condition and medical history and decide on the type of anesthesia that's right for you.

Intravenous fluids will be started by a nurse or by your anesthesiologist. The intravenous line, or IV, is crucial to your anesthesia. It is through the IV line that the anesthesiologist will give you the medications and fluids needed to keep you comfortable and safe.

Often, you will receive some preoperative sedatives to relax you before you enter the operating room.

In the Operating Room Once you are in the operating room, all the monitors will be attached. Three sticky pads will be placed on your shoulders and side for the electrocardiogram. A blood pressure cuff will be wrapped around your arm or leg. The pulse oximeter will be attached to a fingertip.

If you are having general anesthesia, the anesthesiologist will inject some medication through the intravenous line.

In a few seconds, you will drift off to sleep. You will not be aware of anything that happens in the operating room.

Anesthesia is a continuous process, not a single shot of medication that knocks you out. For as long as is required by the surgeon, the anesthesiologist administers varying amounts of medication and fluids according to the needs of the surgeon, the type and length of the operation, your weight and age and your vital signs.

Sometimes, to help the surgeon operate, you will be given medication that causes profound muscle relaxation. In this case, you will not breathe for yourself. The anesthesiologist ensures that you get the oxygen you need by placing a tube in your windpipe and attaching the tube to a mechanical ventilator.

When surgery is complete, the anesthesiologist will reverse the anesthesia and you will be transported to the recovery room to slowly wake up.

WHEN YOU WAKE UP

Waking up from anesthesia is not much different than waking up from any other sleep. The newer anesthetic agents have remarkably few side effects, so you may or may not feel nauseated. Vomiting is rare.

You will be closely monitored by specialized recovery room staff until you are alert enough to be transferred to the same-day surgery area. There you may be with your family or friends until you recover fully. You will be given something light to eat and drink, then be discharged home. Be sure to make arrangements beforehand to have someone drive you home after surgery and, if possible, to stay with you for 24 hours.

Pain How much pain you experience after the operation depends on the type of surgery you have. Any operation that involves cutting through the skin will leave you with an incision that will cause discomfort for a few days.

As you wake up, the anesthesiologist will administer intravenous pain relievers so you will be comfortable in the recovery room. As these wear off, you may require an injection or oral pain relievers. Your surgeon will provide you with a prescription for pain relievers to take when you get home.

At Home Although anesthetic agents wear off quickly these days, microscopic amounts of medication remain in your bloodstream for many hours. You may experience a little residual tiredness or nausea, but this should pass after the first day home.

◆ You should not drive a car, operate heavy machinery or make any important decisions for at least 24 hours after you have received anesthesia.

◆ Do not drink alcohol or take any medications except those prescribed for you.

CHILDREN AND ANESTHESIA

The only thing that provokes more anxiety than having surgery yourself is the prospect of your child going through the same process (*see* Chapter 4). As the old saying goes, "It's not just the child having surgery, it's the entire family." There are many small operations, but there is no such thing as a small anesthetic.

Besides guiding your child safely through the surgery and anesthesia, the role of the anesthesiologist is to provide comfort to the whole family. And the key to feeling comfortable is to be well informed.

Speak to your child's anesthesiologist beforehand. Ask as many questions as you need to understand fully the sequence of events you and your child will be going through. Then talk honestly with your child about what to expect. Explain that she or he will be in an unfamiliar place but that there will be many friendly doctors and nurses around to help. Tell your child that you will remain nearby for almost the entire time and that you will be there soon after she or he wakes up.

Dealing with Separation Every effort is made to have at least one parent accompany the child for as long as possible, but at some point, the child must go into the operating room without mom or dad. Children at a cooperative age (usually five and up) can accompany the anesthesiologist to the operating room.

If your child is too frightened to separate easily, a sedative can be given while you are still in the preoperative room. This sedative could be a small injection or a rectal suppository. Only after the child gets drowsy will he or she be taken to the operating room. This will avoid one of the major traumas of the day because your child will have no memory of being separated from you.

In the Operating Room Anesthesia in adults is usually induced by injecting medication into the intravenous line, but it is sometimes difficult, even traumatic, to start an IV line in a child. It is common to offer a soft plastic breathing mask that covers the nose and mouth.

The child is asked to breathe in and out slowly. Anesthetic vapors are mixed with oxygen and the child smoothly falls to sleep. All needles are avoided and the intravenous is started after the child is asleep.

Some surgical centers allow one parent to accompany the child to the operating room to make this inhalation induction a little easier, but this has to be discussed with your anesthesiologist ahead of time.

In the Recovery Room Parents are usually not allowed in the recovery room

because the staff and anesthesiologist will be quite busy attending to the immediate needs of the awakening patient. Your child will still be groggy and will not even realize that you're not there. As soon as the child becomes more alert, she or he will be taken to the outpatient surgical area to recover more fully with you and other members of the family.

After the Operation It is normal for your child to be arousable but sleepy for a few hours.
◆ Expect a day of crankiness.
◆ Your child may or may not vomit; either is normal.
◆ Appetite will return in time, but don't be in a hurry to feed your child. He or she will have already received adequate fluids through the IV line.
◆ Depending on the surgery performed, there may be some pain that can be treated with an injection or a Tylenol suppository.
◆ Your child will quickly return to normal over the next 24 hours, but if you have any questions do not hesitate to call the outpatient surgery center, the anesthesiologist or the surgeon at any time.

QUESTIONS TO ASK YOUR ANESTHESIOLOGIST
◆ What are your qualifications? Are you Board-certified?
◆ What is the best anesthesia for me for this type of surgery?
◆ What are the side effects?
◆ How will I feel when I wake up? Will I be in pain?
◆ How will my pain be treated?
◆ When can I eat or drink?
◆ When can I go home?
◆ Is there anything special that I should do or avoid doing at home?
◆ Who should I call if I have a problem?

6
SKIN CONDITIONS AND BIOPSY PROCEDURES

Robert E. Allen Jr., MD, FACS

———————◇———————

Most conditions of the skin and of the tissues just beneath the skin (subcutaneous) can be surgically managed effectively on an outpatient basis. Most of the procedures can be performed under local anesthesia, but premedication and general anesthesia may be used instead if you feel any anxiety about the surgery after your surgeon explains the details.

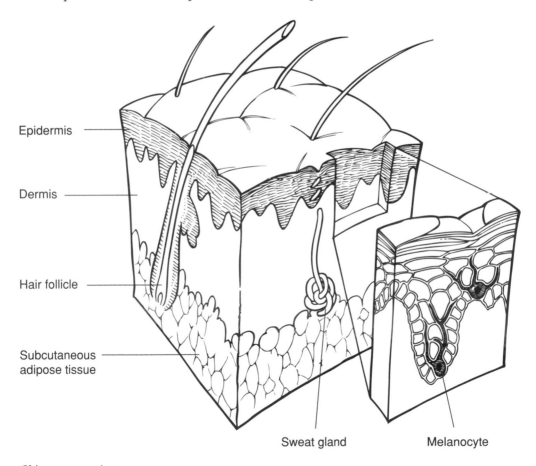

Epidermis

Dermis

Hair follicle

Subcutaneous adipose tissue

Sweat gland

Melanocyte

Skin cross-section

MOLES AND SPOTS

Moles are composed of pigment-producing cells called melanocytes. In normal skin, melanocytes appear as clear cells in the uppermost layer of the skin, the epidermis. These may increase in number in the various layers of the skin to form harmless pigmented spots.

◆ Freckles (lentigo) are accumulations of melanocytes within the lower layer of the epidermis (the basal layer).

◆ Other forms of moles occur in the layers of the skin where the dermis and epidermis meet. These moles vary from simple flat spots to raised masses of tissue. These simple moles occur anywhere in the skin, including the nail beds. They are occasionally seen in the thin mucous membrane covering most of the eyeball and lining the eyelids (the conjunctiva), but are rare in other mucous membranes.

◆ The blue mole is a tumor composed of melanocytes that occurs most commonly on the face, the back of the hand and the top of the foot and on the lower back in certain races (Mongolian blue spot). The blue mole is very darkly pigmented, but because of the overlying layer of normal and sometimes thin epidermis, it looks shiny blue or slate gray. Malignant changes are exceptionally rare.

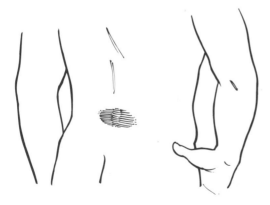

Mongolian blue spot

◆ More than 95 percent of adults have one or more darkly pigmented brownish red spots called nevi. They may have a scalloped appearance and may have hair growing out of them. Large nevi that are present from birth (congenital) may carry an increased risk of malignant change.

When Moles Should Be Removed
Most moles cause no problems and generally are not treated. But treatment may be required if they cause cosmetic problems, if they are in an area where they are subjected to repeated injury, such as being continually cut when shaving, or if there is any suggestion that malignant change has occurred.

A mole should always be removed when it shows evidence of change or new growth. Variation in color, especially a darkening of the mole, an increase in size, irregular borders, itching and ulceration all indicate that the mole should be treated.

The only effective treatment is surgical removal, and all the tissues removed must be sent to a pathologist for histologic examination.

Surgical Procedure A mole should be removed with an excisional biopsy. An elliptical incision is made and the entire lesion is removed, rather than a small piece of it. A small rim of normal tissue around the mole and a small part of the subcutaneous tissue are also taken.

A shaved biopsy—in which a scalpel is used to remove a thin slice of tissue—is not recommended. If the lesion turns out to be a melanoma, pathologic interpretation is difficult if the lesion is not completely excised. Melanomas can spread deeply into the layers of the skin, and with a shaved biopsy the depth of invasion cannot be determined. The depth of invasion helps determine both the prognosis for cure and the planning of adequate treatment.

In most cases, the wound is simply

closed with stitches and a dressing is applied.

After the Operation Wounds will heal very quickly.
◆ Pain is minimal after the first 24 hours and the risk of infection is low.
◆ Pathologic results should be available in one to three days, depending on the size of the lesion and the number of lesions removed.
◆ Stitches will stay in place for five to 10 days, depending on where the mole was and how much tension is put on the incision. Wounds on the back, for example, tend to heal more slowly than wounds on the neck.

MALIGNANT MELANOMA

Malignant melanoma is a cancer that arises from the melanocytes in the epidermis. It is the most dangerous form of skin cancer and can spread to most of the body's organs and tissues.

The rate of increase in the incidence of malignant melanoma is greater than that for any other cancer. Its incidence has doubled every 10 years in countries close to the equator and every 10 to 15 years in more temperate zones.

Increased exposure to sunlight is mainly responsible for this rapid increase.

About 60 percent of all melanomas occur in pre-existing moles. Again, signs of malignant changes include changes in size, irregularity in contour, variation in color, itching and ulceration.

Types of Melanoma There are four clinical types of melanoma: lentigo maligna, superficial spreading, nodular and acral-lentiginous.

The measured depth of invasion of the tumor into the various levels of the skin is the most important indicator used by a clinical pathologist to correlate the pathology of the specimen and the prognosis for cure or recurrence. But the thickness of the tumor is a better measure of prognosis than the level of invasion.

Surgical Procedure The only curative treatment for melanoma is the surgical removal of the tumor along with an adequate margin of normal skin. Again, shaved biopsies should be avoided. In the first instance, the tumor and a small amount of skin are removed because surgeons are reluctant to remove a large area of skin until a definite diagnosis is made.

Once the diagnosis of melanoma is confirmed, the surgeon will recommend that a larger area of skin be removed, constituting an adequate excision. One problem has been defining what "adequate" means. For low-risk and intermediate-risk lesions—thin tumors or those of medium thickness—1/2 to 3/4 in. (1 to 2 cm) are adequate margins. For thicker, high-risk lesions, a margin of 1 in. (2.5 cm) is adequate in most cases.

After the lesion is removed, the resulting wound may be closed by stretching the skin and stitching the edges together. But when a large area of skin has been removed, the remaining skin may need to be freed up from the

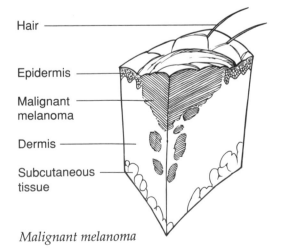

Hair

Epidermis

Malignant melanoma

Dermis

Subcutaneous tissue

Malignant melanoma

underlying tissue so that it will pull together. This can create a large potential space underneath the skin flaps. Some surgeons may place a temporary tube into this space so that fluid collecting in the space can be drained.

In a few cases, it will not be possible to bring the skin back together, so a skin graft will be performed. A thin piece of skin will be removed from the upper leg or buttock and placed over the wound. The skin at the donor site will heal by regeneration. Within a few days, the skin graft will attach to the wound and begin to grow.

The entire specimen of the melanoma and the margins should be sent for pathological study so that proper treatment can be planned.

When there is evidence of tumor spread to the lymph nodes or distant sites such as the lungs and liver, the lymph nodes and metastases may also be surgically removed, but these procedures are not performed on an outpatient basis.

After the Operation When larger amounts of skin are removed, the risks of bleeding and of fluid collecting underneath the skin are greater.

◆ Stitches are often left in longer than usual because of increased tension on the skin edges.

◆ Skin grafts will require extra care and protection until the graft is firmly attached.

NON-MELANOMA SKIN CANCERS

Skin cancer is the most common form of cancer, and the incidence of all forms of the disease is increasing. The annual incidence of non-melanoma skin cancer in the United States is 160 per 100,000 population.

There are several proven causes of non-melanoma skin cancer, including increased exposure to sunlight (ultraviolet light), ionizing radiation, a deficiency or suppression of the immune system and exposure to cancer-causing chemicals (carcinogens). The most potent of the chemical carcinogens are polycyclic hydrocarbons. These excite the development of procarcinogens, which ultimately become the carcinogens directly causing malignant cell transformation. Of all these causes, increased exposure to sunlight is probably the most significant.

There are two major types of non-melanoma skin cancer.

Basal Cell Carcinoma Basal cell carcinoma (also called rodent ulcer and basal cell epithelioma) is a malignant tumor arising from the basal layer of the epidermis, the hair follicles and the skin glands. It is the most common form of skin cancer by far. It is a disease of old people and is more frequently found in men than women. Exposure to sunlight is a predisposing factor and it is very common in Caucasians living in temperate and tropical climates.

Ninety percent of basal cell carcinomas are found on the face, usually above a line running from the lobe of the ear to the corner of the mouth. The most common site is around the inner corner of the eye. The common types are nodular, cystic and ulcerated.

Basal cell carcinomas have a great diversity of appearance (the tumor, along with syphilis, is known as the great imitator). Although often called a rodent ulcer, many of the lesions are non-ulcerated and have a nodular appearance, with a pearly or dark translucent color. It often looks as if it contains water with a network of fiery red blood vessels on the surface.

It is usually diagnosed when someone sees his or her doctor about a "spot that never heals."

Surgical Procedure: Basal Cell Carcinomas Basal cell carcinomas are radiosensitive and can be adequately treated with radiotherapy, but they are best treated with surgical excision. Surgical treatment is usually curative.

Excision with subsequent closure of the skin edges is possible in most cases. Where large areas of skin are removed, a skin graft may be necessary. In the hands of an expert surgeon, the cosmetic results after removal are usually acceptable. Examination of the specimen allows the pathologist to confirm that the cancer has been completely removed.

Squamous Cell Carcinomas These cancers arise within the epidermis or the other cells in the skin that produce keratin. This type of skin cancer is less common than basal cell carcinoma, but is more malignant and grows more rapidly.

Squamous cell carcinoma occurs in skin that has been exposed to tropical sunlight for many years. Sun damage becomes evident after 10 to 20 years, so squamous cell carcinoma tends to occur in later life, increasing after the age of 60. It can appear for the first time in the normal facial skin of elderly people, but occurs more often in pre-existing skin lesions or in areas of the skin that have been exposed to radiation.

Squamous cell carcinoma is uncommon in dark-skinned people and is most common in people of Celtic origin living in sunny climates. There is a high incidence in albino members of dark-skinned races.

Some environmental carcinogens may be responsible for this condition, but the single most common cause is exposure to sunlight. Squamous cell carcinoma does not usually arise from healthy-looking skin.

The first clinical sign of malignancy may be a thickening of the skin area, an area raised from the surface or an ulceration, but in all cases the lesion is firm.

The tissue around the growth is red and the edges around it are a dirty yellowish red. The common sites are those most exposed to the sun—the backs of the hands, forearms, the upper part of the face and, in males especially, the lower lip and the ear.

Surgical Procedure: Squamous Cell Carcinoma The best treatment for this type of skin cancer is also surgical excision. If the lesion is small, an excisional biopsy may possibly be curative. The surgeon will attempt to achieve an excision with at least a 1/2 to 3/4 in. (1 to 2 cm) margin of skin around the tumor.

Squamous cell carcinoma of the skin rarely spreads to the lymph nodes, so a prophylactic lymph node dissection is not necessary.

After the Operation Surgery for both basal cell and squamous cell carcinomas usually involves removing only very small areas of tissue, and postoperative complications are unusual. In the rare cases of larger lesions, potential complications are the same as those for melanoma surgery.
- When larger amounts of skin are removed, the risks of bleeding and of fluid collecting underneath the skin are greater.
- Stitches are often left in longer than usual because of increased tension on the skin edges.
- Skin grafts will require extra care and protection until the graft is firmly attached.

CYSTS

Cysts are fluid-filled sacs of tissue found in many parts of the body. Most cysts found in the skin are epidermoid cysts with an epithelial lining. They are referred to as sebaceous cysts, named after the sebaceous glands that produce sebum, a substance that lubricates the skin and keeps it supple. Most of these cysts are benign and usually have no malignant potential, but they tend to become infected if injured. If a cyst does become infected, most surgeons won't remove it until the infection has completely cleared.

Surgical Procedure The standard treatment is excision of the cyst and the complete excision of the epithelial lining. If the epithelial lining is not removed, the cyst tends to recur. The area is closed with sutures.

After the Operation If the cyst has been infected in the past, there is a slightly increased risk that the wound could become infected.

◆ If you notice pain, warmth and/or redness, contact your surgeon so that appropriate treatment can be given.

LIPOMAS

A lipoma is a slow-growing tumor composed of adult fat cells. They may be small and oval or large with many finger-like projections. They occur anywhere in the body where fat is found. The head and neck area, abdominal wall and the thighs are particularly favored sites. Subcutaneous lipomas are commonly found on the shoulders or the back, although no part of the body is immune. Multiple lipomas are not uncommon.

Lipomas are usually benign but can undergo malignant changes. Large lipomas, particularly those changing in size, shape or consistency, should be removed, but small ones that do not change size need not be treated at all. If a lipoma is causing trouble because of its size, site or appearance or because of pain, it should be excised.

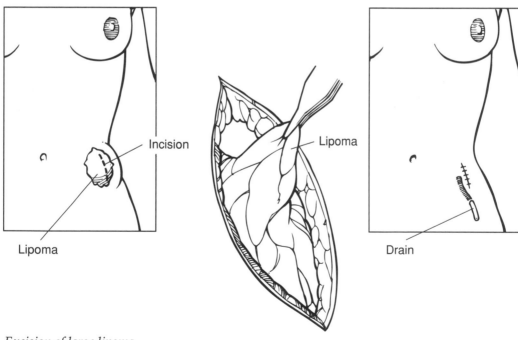

Excision of large lipoma

Surgical Procedure During the operation, any finger-like projections of the tumor into the surrounding tissue are also excised. If all of it is not removed, the lipoma may return. The incision is usually closed with stitches.

After the Operation In some cases, there will be a large space left after the operation. A drain may be required to remove the fluid that will collect in the space and to allow healing to proceed. (*See* Malignant Melanoma, "Surgical Procedure.")

MUSCLE BIOPSIES

Muscle biopsies are often performed to discover the cause of unexplained muscle weakness. What might be found is evidence of immune system disorders or degenerative diseases such as muscular dystrophy.

Surgical Procedure The incision for a muscle biopsy is usually small. A small plastic clamp is used to keep the muscle from contracting and a small piece of the muscle is removed. The ideal specimen for analysis is usually about 3/4 in. by 1/2 in. (2 cm by 1 cm), taken along the long axis of the muscle. The specimen should be sent to pathology fresh in saline so that special studies can be performed.

The incision is usually closed with stitches.

After the Operation The wound from the biopsy tends to heal rapidly and infection is uncommon.

QUESTIONS TO ASK YOUR SURGEON

◆ After the skin biopsy, will I need additional surgery?
◆ What are the chances that the skin lesions will be a cancer?
◆ What is the relative effectiveness of various types of treatment for skin cancers?
◆ Are there alternative forms of treatment for my cancer, such as radiation?

7
BREAST SURGERY

Stanley P.L. Leong, MD, FACS, *and James R. Macho,* MD, FACS

Other than cosmetic procedures performed by plastic surgeons (*see* Chapter 14), almost all outpatient surgery to the breast is done to diagnose or treat breast cancer. These procedures commonly involve removing lumps that can be felt or are identified on a mammogram (lumpectomy) or removing a section of the breast (quadrantectomy).

WEIGHING THE RISKS OF BREAST CANCER

Women are becoming very aware of the risk of breast cancer. The statistics are that one in nine women will develop breast cancer over a lifetime estimated at 85 years. What the statistics don't tell is that most women who develop the disease are older rather than young, with the average age being around 60, and that in many cases the breast cancer will be a treatable chronic problem but will not cause death.

Risk Factors Some women are at higher risk than others for developing breast cancer. For this reason, surgeons tend to ask many questions when evaluating women with breast problems. The most significant risk factors are:
◆ Increasing age.
◆ A family history of breast cancer, especially among mothers, sisters and daughters.
◆ The early onset of menstruation.
◆ First pregnancy after age 30.
◆ Late menopause.

All women, especially those with high risk factors, should be evaluated regularly. A thorough breast examination should be part of every gynecologic examination and be part of every regular physical. In most cases, the chances for a cure and a life without cancer are high if a cancer is found early.

Breast Self-Examination Understanding the need for and practicing breast self-examination help a woman increase her chances of detecting breast cancer in its early stages.

After puberty, every woman should systematically examine her breasts every month, following the techniques recommended by the American Cancer Society. Self-examination picks up a significant percentage of breast lesions.

Screening Mammography One of the reasons for the increased statistical incidence of breast cancer may be that more lesions are being recognized by screening mammography. This technique has been used much more extensively in the past few years than it was a decade ago.

Screening mammography, however, picks up benign lesions as well as cancerous ones. In most cases, the lesion cannot be diagnosed conclusively on the basis of the mammogram alone, so a biopsy must be done to determine whether a breast lesion is benign or malignant.

The American Cancer Society recommends that all women have a baseline

CANADIAN BREAST CANCER FOUNDATION

MONTHLY BREAST SELF-EXAM

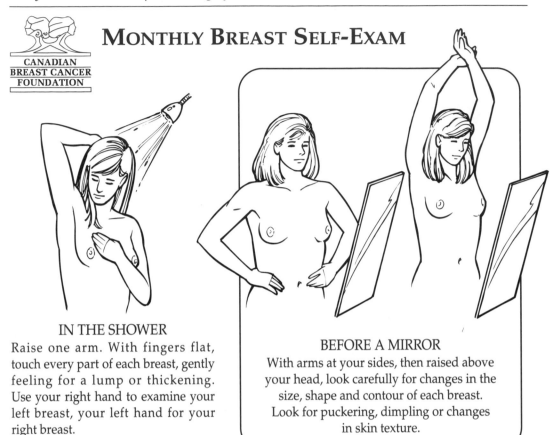

IN THE SHOWER
Raise one arm. With fingers flat, touch every part of each breast, gently feeling for a lump or thickening. Use your right hand to examine your left breast, your left hand for your right breast.

BEFORE A MIRROR
With arms at your sides, then raised above your head, look carefully for changes in the size, shape and contour of each breast. Look for puckering, dimpling or changes in skin texture.

LYING DOWN
Fingers flat, press gently in small circles, starting at the outermost top edge of your breast and spiraling in toward the nipple. Examine every part of the breast. Repeat with the other breast.

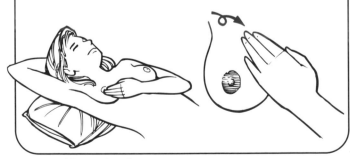

With your arm resting on a firm surface, use the same circular motion to examine the underarm area. This is breast tissue, too. Gently squeeze both nipples and look for discharge.

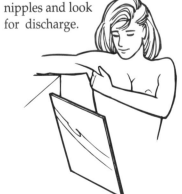

Breast self-examination

mammogram at age 40. Change in a mammogram is very important in assessing a new growth or lesion. Any woman who has significant risk factors for breast cancer should have a yearly mammogram for the rest of her life. If she is not in a high-risk category, she may need a mammogram only every two years until age 50.

After age 50, all women should have a mammogram every year. This recommendation is based on the fact that early detection of breast cancer by mammography may result in better control and potential cure of the disease. Most women treated for early breast cancer will be free of the disease for the rest of their lives.

Biopsy A surgeon has no way of knowing whether a lump is cancer without taking a piece of the mass and examining it under a microscope. So when you, your physician or a health worker discover a lump, it should be biopsied. If the lump can be felt, an open biopsy is performed. When the lump is discovered only by mammogram, a needle localization approach is used. Both procedures may be done in an outpatient setting.

Only about 20 percent of all biopsies are cancerous. In women aged 35 to 39, the ratio of benign to malignant lesions is about 17 to 1. Between 50 and 54, the ratio becomes 5 to 1. Between ages 70 and 74, the ratio is 3 to 1.

Histologic Diagnosis of the Biopsy Specimen The most important information obtained from a biopsy is the microscopic tissue diagnosis based on the examination by a pathologist.

If the lesion is benign, nothing else needs to be done, although you may need to see your physician at regular intervals. This is especially important if the diagnosis is such that there are greater risks of developing breast cancer in the future.

If the lesion is malignant, additional surgery is needed to make sure that the adjacent tissues (margins) are clear of cancer cells.

DISCUSSING TREATMENT OPTIONS WITH YOUR SURGEON

Surgeons dealing with a breast problem generally do not let the diagnosis and treatment process drag out. They realize that the possibility of cancer creates a very emotional and fearful situation. Usually, a lump can be removed easily and the diagnosis obtained quickly, so surgeons will try to schedule surgery soon after a potentially cancerous mass is discovered.

When a diagnosis of cancer is made, various treatment options may be considered. Treatment may involve lumpectomy, axillary lymph node dissection plus postoperative radiation therapy, or a modified radical mastectomy. Discuss each of these options in detail with your surgeon, listen to his or her recommendation and perhaps get one or more second opinions from other physicians.

The best therapeutic choice will depend on your age, the size, location and stage of the tumor, whether there is evidence of spread to the lymph nodes in the armpit (axillary lymph nodes) and whether radiation therapy is easily obtainable.

Personal preferences are also important. There are aesthetic, practical and psychological considerations. Waiting two weeks or even a month after diagnosis before further surgery makes no difference to the prognosis, so consider all options carefully before making your decision.

NEEDLE BIOPSIES

Two kinds of needles are used to biopsy a breast lump.

◆ A fine needle, very much like the one used for drawing blood, is used to draw out some cells from the lump for examination on a slide. This is called a fine needle aspiration.

If the lump is a cyst, this is a useful procedure. The fluid is aspirated and the lump will disappear. If the mass does not return, no further biopsy is needed. If the mass is solid, the needle can be used to obtain cells from the mass.

◆ A larger needle is used to remove a small piece of the lump for examination under the microscope. This is called a core biopsy because a small cylinder of tissue is removed for examination.

Your surgeon may recommend an open biopsy if the needle biopsy is negative. The problem with all needle biopsies is that they remove only a small piece of a lump. The area of cancer in a lump may be quite small and the rest of the lump may be due to the swelling and scarring of the surrounding tissues. If cancer cells are found on a needle biopsy, this procedure is very helpful. However, there is also a chance that the needle might miss the area of the cancer. Therefore, a negative result does not eliminate the possibility that a cancer is present. In fact, there is a 15 to 25 percent chance that a cancer may be found on an open biopsy performed after a negative needle biopsy.

Your surgeon may decide to remove a lump without performing a needle biopsy if the likelihood of a positive result is low and if the lump will need to be removed regardless of the biopsy result.

OPEN BIOPSIES

Two types of open biopsies are done.
◆ An incisional biopsy removes a portion of the lump. This method is used when the mass is large and surgery may be more involved after microscopic diagnosis.

◆ An excisional biopsy means that the entire lump is removed. This technique is generally used for smaller lesions. If the lesion proves to be benign, no further surgery is needed.

After either of these procedures, you will have a permanent scar, although the cosmetic defect may be slight. Discuss with your surgeon what type of incision she or he will make.

Surgical Procedure Both open biopsy procedures may be done as outpatient procedures, with a local anesthetic such as lidocaine to minimize pain. This procedure is much like the injection you are given in a dentist's office before having a cavity filled.

The procedure may take about an hour. Older women are monitored by electrocardiogram.
◆ If the lump is in the upper half of the breast, a curved horizontal incision is usually made.
◆ If the lesion is close to the nipple, an incision may be made along the edge of the areola or nipple to minimize scarring.
◆ If the lesion is in the lower half of the breast, the surgeon may make a diagonal incision.

The incision carries down through the skin and into the fatty tissue, then around the area of the lump. Before being sent to a pathologist for examination and diagnosis, the tissue specimen is marked by stitches to indicate its position in the breast.

Any bleeding from small vessels will be stopped by electrocoagulation. This involves passing an electric current through the site of the bleeding, so if you are having a local anesthetic, you might feel some mild discomfort, especially if the lump is close to the muscle.

Your surgeon will usually inject some local anesthetic in the area before beginning electrocoagulation. Direct

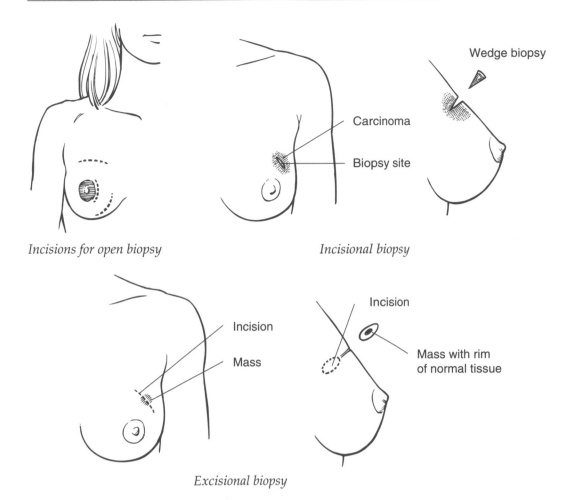

Incisions for open biopsy　　　　　*Incisional biopsy*

Wedge biopsy

Carcinoma

Biopsy site

Incision

Mass

Incision

Mass with rim
of normal tissue

Excisional biopsy

communication between patient and surgeon is important during such a procedure, so if you feel any discomfort or pain, let the surgeon know right away. The area can be anesthetized further.

Usually, only the skin is closed so that there will not be any deformity to dimple the breast skin. The space left after the biopsy will be filled in by the surrounding tissue, and no significant defect will be noticed.

A drain (a small plastic tube) may be left in the wound if there is a large defect. Drains are usually not necessary when the defect is small.

The skin is usually closed with what

is called subcuticular stitching. This involves a cosmetic type of closure, with the stitches under the skin rather than through it. This prevents railroad-track scarring and leaves a very fine scar line. Dissolving stitches are often used so that no separate procedure is needed to remove them.

After the Operation The procedure is usually performed without any significant complications, and the wound heals very nicely.
◆ There is minimal (less than 2 percent) risk of infection.
◆ If the bleeding is not carefully and

thoroughly stopped during the operation, there is a chance of blood clots forming within the wound (hematoma). The clot is usually left alone and will be absorbed by the body. If the hematoma is infected, however, an additional procedure will be needed to remove it.

NEEDLE LOCALIZATION BIOPSY

This procedure, which is similar to an open biopsy, may be necessary because the lump has been detected on a mammogram but cannot be felt.

Surgical Procedure In a radiology department, a radiologist inserts a needle into the breast, aimed at the mammographic position of the lump. The end of the needle, which is opened like a fish hook, becomes securely anchored to the lump.

In the operating room, the surgeon cuts toward this area so that the lump localized by the tip of the needle can be successfully removed. The wound is closed in the same way as in an open biopsy.

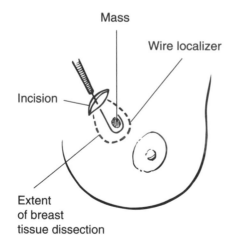

Needle localization biopsy

STEREOTACTIC BREAST BIOPSY

In this newer method of diagnosing breast cancer, no open biopsy is needed.

Surgical Procedure The breast is rested on a table with an opening. The breast is positioned through the opening so that it dangles somewhat beneath the table. A mammogram is taken to determine the position of the lesion.

Guided by computer-assisted x-rays, a radiologist inserts a specialized needle into the breast and removes a 1 to 2 mm portion of the lesion.

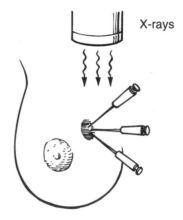

Stereotactic breast biopsy with mammogram

Multiple biopsies may done to secure a good sampling of the area for an accurate diagnosis.

There is evidence that the results of this procedure are very reliable. In some situations, the open biopsy may not be needed before making a diagnosis and planning further treatment.

LUMPECTOMY

A lumpectomy is the removal of the lump and its surrounding tissue (margins).

Surgical Procedure A lumpectomy is done under local anesthesia in the same way as an open biopsy, except that a more generous amount of normal tissue is removed.

As in an open biopsy, stitches are used to indicate the position of the removed tissue specimen within the breast. This is done so that the pathologist examining the specimen can determine whether the margins are clear of cancer.

If the lesion shows invasive cancer, the lymph nodes may have to be removed for staging. The stage of cancer is defined by the size of the tumor, whether lymph nodes are involved and whether tumor cells have spread to other parts of the body. Staging determines whether chemotherapy should be given after surgery.

LYMPH NODE REMOVAL

It used to be thought that the lymph nodes in the armpit should be removed because cancer cells spread to these lymph nodes first and the surgeon wanted to be sure all the cancer was removed. Today, the lymph nodes are usually removed because they are a good indicator of the prognosis.

If the lymph nodes are all negative for cancer, the patient will probably do very well because there is less of a chance that the cancer has spread to the far areas of the body.

If the lymph nodes are filled with cancer, it is more likely that the cancer has spread to other areas. This helps the surgeon decide on the most appropriate type of therapy.

Surgical Procedure A lymph node dissection is usually performed under general anesthesia, and may be done as an outpatient procedure.

An incision is made underneath the armpit and the axillary lymph nodes are removed.

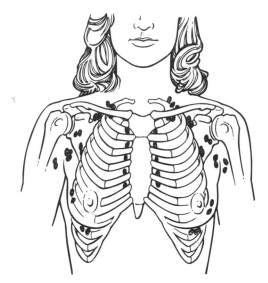

Location of lymph nodes

After the Operation You will experience some numbness in the shoulder and the upper arm for the first few days.

◆ There is a possibility of fluid collecting in the armpit after surgery, so a drain (a small plastic tube) is usually inserted. The skin flaps heal onto the underlying tissue while the space is adequately drained. The drain stays in the armpit for about a week until the drainage becomes minimal.

◆ If the lymph nodes are positive, you will receive chemotherapy after surgery.

◆ Radiation will be given to the entire breast if only lumpectomy is performed. Lumpectomy plus local radiation to the breast and removal of axillary lymph nodes is equivalent to a modified radical mastectomy.

MODIFIED RADICAL MASTECTOMY

A modified radical mastectomy is the removal of the entire breast and the axillary lymph nodes. What distinguishes this from the traditional Halsted radical mastectomy is that in this procedure, no chest muscles are removed.

A modified radical mastectomy is generally done when the tumor is large and the breast is small. This approach may also be used for women who refuse to have radiation treatment or who do not have easy access to radiology facilities.

Surgical Procedure A modified radical mastectomy is performed under general anesthesia. Some centers perform the operation as an outpatient procedure only for a few select patients. Women are usually admitted to the hospital for a day or two for observation.

FOLLOW-UP
After any of these treatments, careful follow-up is essential. Your response to treatment will be monitored and any recurrence of the cancer will be detected.

Follow-up involves regular physical examinations and mammograms, blood tests, imaging studies such as x-rays or CT scans, and other specialized procedures.

QUESTIONS TO ASK YOUR SURGEON
◆ What is the risk of my having breast cancer?
◆ When will I be informed of the biopsy result?
◆ Will stitches need to be removed?
◆ If cancer is present, can it be treated with lumpectomy, axillary lymph node removal or radiation therapy?
◆ Will I need chemotherapy?
◆ If mastectomy is performed, what are my choices for reconstruction?
◆ What additional tests will be required?
◆ How often will I have to be examined after treatment?
◆ What are the risks of developing a second breast cancer?

8
ABDOMEN

Allan Siperstein, MD, FACS, *and James R. Macho,* MD, FACS

———————◇———————

Until a few years ago, almost all abdominal operations were performed using conventional, or open, surgical techniques. The surgeon would make a 6 to 8 in. (15 to 20 cm) incision through the abdominal wall, an incision large enough that the surgeon's hands and the surgical instruments would have access to the area being treated.

Such operations involve several days of hospitalization and an extensive recovery time, because what determines recovery is the incision itself rather than the procedures performed inside the body. When a muscle is cut over a distance of several inches, many nerve endings are cut and there is much pulling of the abdominal wall around the edges of the surgical wound as a patient moves about after an operation.

For patients undergoing open surgical procedures, surgeons recommend waiting at least six weeks before performing any strenuous physical or lifting activities to allow time for the incision to heal. Failure to heed this warning could result in a weakening of the wound and the later development of a hernia. Even if the wound heals normally, a patient undergoing open surgery will be left with a large scar as a life-long reminder of the procedure.

In the 1980s, a new and less invasive approach was developed for several of the most common abdominal operations.

LAPAROSCOPIC TECHNIQUES

Laparoscopic surgery—or minimally invasive surgery, as it is sometimes called—is performed by operating with long, thin instruments passed through small incisions in the abdominal wall. The instruments are operated by the surgeon's hands, which remain outside the patient's body.

As the surgeon cannot look directly into the abdomen, the organs and tissues are seen via a laparoscope, a 1/2 in. (1 cm) diameter scope with a small camera attached that is passed into the belly. The surgeon and other members of the operating team view the area being treated on a video monitor.

To provide room to maneuver in the belly, the abdominal cavity is inflated with carbon dioxide gas. Under these conditions, general anesthesia is usually required, since the inflation of the abdomen makes normal breathing difficult. The gas puts considerable pressure on the diaphragm.

Many different instruments are used in laparoscopic surgery, and newer ones are being developed. In the early days of this technique, there was much enthusiasm about using a surgical laser to accomplish some of the internal procedures. It has now been shown that the standard electrocautery, which heats and seals the blood vessels, is much easier and cheaper to use than the laser, and involves much less blood loss. Most surgeons who initially championed the laser have now abandoned the technique.

Advantages Laparoscopic surgery is a true advance in the field of surgery. Just as the development of anesthesia allowed surgical procedures to be performed safely and without pain, laparoscopic surgery results in less pain and a much faster recovery.

As the techniques developed, surgeons were amazed to see that patients undergoing, for example, laparoscopic removal of the gallbladder could usually eat on the evening of surgery and could be discharged home the next day with minimal discomfort. Patients having a conventional open removal of the gallbladder often require four days of hospitalization.

There are several other advantages of laparoscopic surgery.
◆ Less postoperative pain means that patients require fewer narcotics for pain control and so tend to be less drowsy once the anesthetics used during the operation wear off. Narcotics also tend to make people nauseated. The combination of less pain and fewer nauseating narcotic side effects contributes to patients returning to their normal eating habits more quickly.
◆ Smaller incisions that tend to heal rapidly mean that patients are often able to return to work within a week.
◆ Smaller incisions also produce a markedly improved cosmetic result, with several small scars that may disappear altogether rather than one large scar that is visible for life.

Further advances in laparoscopic surgery make it possible for other commonly performed surgical procedures to be done on an outpatient basis (*see also* Chapter 17, "Gynecologic Surgery," and Chapter 18, "Urologic Surgery").

THE LAPAROSCOPIC SURGEON

General surgeons who perform laparoscopic surgery take advanced training to learn the skills involved. This usually involves several days of lectures and practical experience in performing such procedures on anesthetized animals. After completing these courses, surgeons must then perform five to 10 of these procedures with an experienced laparoscopic surgeon before they are allowed to perform the procedures independently.

It is very important for a surgeon to be thoroughly trained before using laparoscopic tools and techniques. In the hands of an inexperienced person, serious complications can develop.
◆ Because the field of vision is limited through the laparoscope, injuries to organs may occur if the instruments are inserted improperly.
◆ If bleeding occurs, it can be difficult to control.
◆ The anatomical structures may appear different through the laparoscope than in open surgery. The surgeon must determine carefully what he or she is cutting to avoid unintentional injury.

When Laparoscopic Surgery May Not Be Appropriate Not all procedures can be performed laparoscopically. But a surgeon may also decide during the operation that it would be unsafe to continue with a laparoscopic approach. This may occur if there is severe scarring within the abdomen, unusual anatomy or unexpected findings. The surgeon may then decide to convert to a standard open operation.

This decision should not be interpreted as a failure on the part of the surgeon. Rather, it may represent good surgical judgment that allows the patient to avoid potentially serious complications, such as an injury to a bile duct.

GALLBLADDER DISEASE

The most common operation performed laparoscopically is removing the gallbladder of someone suffering from symptoms caused by gallstones.

What the Gallbladder Does The liver continuously produces bile, a fluid that aids digestion. The bile passes through a common bile duct from the liver directly into the duodenum, or small intestine. Some of the bile is stored in the gallbladder, a balloon-like sac connected to the common bile duct. After a meal, particularly a meal heavy in fats, the gallbladder contracts, emptying its reserve of digestive fluid into the intestines.

Bile is more than 10 times as concentrated in the gallbladder as it is in the liver. The bile constituents can become supersaturated and crystallize, forming gallstones. They are most commonly composed of cholesterol, with some being made of bilirubinate. Bilirubin is one of the components of hemoglobin excreted in the bile after the breakdown of red blood cells in the liver.

Gallstones are common, especially in women and with advancing age, but most people never experience any symptoms. Others are not so fortunate. Gallstones can produce a variety of symptoms and conditions.

Biliary Colic A gallstone may block the

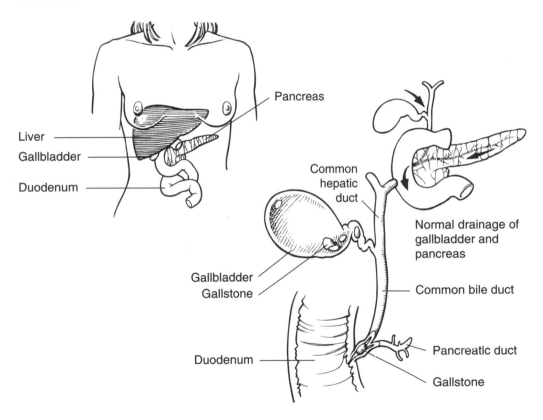

Gallbladder, showing typical places where stones lodge

neck of the gallbladder, not allowing it to contract when stimulated by food in the digestive system. The result is overdistension of the gallbladder and an episode of pain soon after a meal. The pain comes on over several minutes, may persist for 30 minutes to two hours and then subsides spontaneously as the blockage is released. Symptoms disappear almost completely. These painful episodes may occur weeks to months apart.

This condition is termed biliary colic and is experienced as a constant dull pain in the upper right abdomen. Symptoms may include nausea and vomiting as well as abdominal distension.

The symptoms of biliary colic are similar to symptoms caused by ulcer disease, indigestion and gastroenteritis. The pattern of symptoms that makes a physician suspect gallstone disease is that the pain begins about 30 minutes after eating and is especially brought on by fatty foods. Many people suffering from biliary colic tend on their own to avoid fatty foods.

Cholecystitis Should a stone become firmly lodged in the neck of the gallbladder, the pain may persist. If it lasts for a day or more, the diagnosis is acute cholecystitis. Cholecystitis refers to the inflammatory changes of the gallbladder caused by the persistent blockage. The gallbladder may subsequently become infected with bacteria. People suffering from this condition usually have more severe and persistent pain and also often develop a fever.

Blocking Ducts Should a gallstone pass from the gallbladder into the duct leading to the intestine, it may block the duct. It may also block the duct draining the pancreas, which enters the intestine at the same point as the bile duct. Should this happen, the pancreas can

become inflamed (pancreatitis).

Diagnosing Gallstones If the physician suspects that gallstones are a possible cause of abdominal pain, a range of tests may be carried out.

◆ The first test that should be ordered is an ultrasound of the gallbladder to look for stones. This is a non-invasive and inexpensive test and can accurately find the gallstones in about 95 percent of people who have them.

The ultrasound may also reveal evidence of several episodes of biliary colic or acute cholecystitis. The wall of the gallbladder may be thickened or there may be a fluid surrounding the gallbladder because of inflammatory changes.

If the ultrasound shows the presence of gallstones, the physician must then decide whether the stones are the cause of the pain. Some people may have asymptomatic gallstones with a second condition, such as an ulcer disease, that is responsible for their pain.

◆ Blood tests are routinely done to determine whether the liver is functioning normally. An elevated white blood cell count may indicate acute cholecystitis.

◆ The most common of the other tests is a nuclear medicine scan. This test determines whether the gallbladder is functioning normally or whether its duct is blocked by a stone.

Treatment Options Surgery is not usually required when gallstones do not produce symptoms. But for someone who has had several episodes of biliary colic, surgery to remove the gallbladder is usually recommended.

Many patients wonder how they will be able to digest their food without a gallbladder. But some of the function of the gallbladder is taken over by another structure, the common bile duct, when the gallbladder is taken out. People with gallstone disease most often have abnormal gallbladder function to begin with, so these patients are actually able to digest their food better after their gallbladder is removed. There are usually no dietary restrictions, so they can eat whatever they like.

There are other ways to treat gallstones, but none has proved as permanent or effective as removal of the gallbladder.

◆ There are medications that gradually dissolve gallstones, but these are expensive, have several uncomfortable side effects such as diarrhea and are not that effective. In the few cases where the gallstones have actually dissolved, they often returned when the medication was discontinued.

◆ Lithotripsy, a standard treatment for kidney stones that uses sound waves to crush the stones inside the body, has also been tried. Only one patient in 10 is a candidate for biliary lithotripsy because there are many restrictions. In addition, it does not work at all if there are more than three small stones. Patients who have lithotripsy also have to take medicines to dissolve the gallstone fragments. In the few patients who are able to undergo this technique, the success rate is only about 40 percent. This technique, therefore, has been largely abandoned.

Once your physician has decided that surgery is needed, a decision must be made on whether the procedure may be performed laparoscopically. In the past, people who had had previous abdominal operations or who were obese or pregnant were not deemed good candidates for laparoscopic surgery. With experience and advanced equipment, however, such patients are now routinely treated laparoscopically.

People who have acute cholecystitis with greater degrees of inflammation and scarring around the gallbladder make the surgical dissection of the gall-bladder more challenging. But many advanced centers now perform cholecystectomy for acute cholecystitis.

CHOLECYSTECTOMY (REMOVING THE GALLBLADDER)

Although the technical details of a laparoscopic cholecystectomy differ from those in an open cholecystectomy, the amount of internal cutting is similar. The only difference is that whereas the open procedure is performed through a long incision in the abdominal wall, the laparoscopic procedure is performed through four incisions 1/4 to 1/2 in. (5 mm to 1 cm) long.

Before the Operation Preoperative preparation involves a complete history and physical examination, as would be done before any operation.

◆ Routine blood tests are performed.

◆ Only in unusual circumstances would a surgeon request that typed and crossed blood be available for such a procedure. A blood transfusion rarely is required, as only 10 to 20 cc of blood are usually lost.

◆ In older patients, a chest x-ray and electrocardiogram are obtained to make sure there is no underlying cardiac or pulmonary disease.

◆ A general anesthetic is usually given, so you should have nothing to eat or drink after midnight the night before surgery.

Surgical Procedure The operation lasts about an hour. Four small incisions are used to place trocars in the abdominal wall. These are special tubes with valves that allow the abdomen to remain inflated while surgical instruments are inserted and removed. These trocar sites are anesthetized with a long-acting local anesthetic, resulting in very little discomfort after the operation.

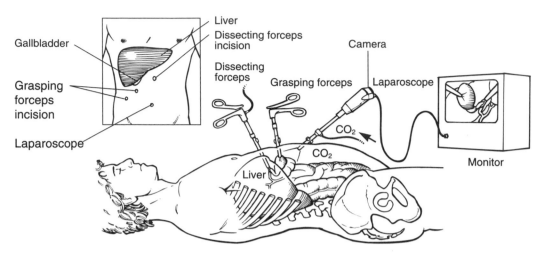

Laparoscopic cholecystectomy

During the procedure, the duct and artery to the gallbladder are carefully identified and divided by stainless steel clips. The gallbladder is then removed from its bed in the liver using the electrocautery. After the gallbladder is completely free, it is removed through one of the tiny incisions.

In some cases, the stones and the gallbladder may be larger than the incision. Part of the gallbladder is then brought out through the skin and opened. Clamps are inserted into the gallbladder to break the stones, then the individual pieces are removed. After the gallblader has been emptied, it can be easily removed.

The abdomen is inspected with the laparoscope to ensure there is no bleeding. The instruments are removed and the carbon dioxide is allowed to escape from the abdominal cavity. The incisions are closed with stitches and usually covered with Band-Aids. Tubes placed during the surgery to drain the stomach and bladder are usually removed before you awaken from the anesthetic.

After the Operation After one to two hours in the recovery room, you will be sent to the ward, where you may resume walking and eating within several hours. In most cases, you will be discharged on the evening of surgery.

◆ There are usually no dietary restrictions after surgery, so you can eat whatever appeals to you.

◆ Non-narcotic pain relievers are usually sufficient to keep you comfortable after surgery.

◆ You can usually resume your normal activities as soon as you are comfortable enough to do so.

◆ Wound infections are uncommon after laparoscopic cholecystectomy, but you should alert your physician if you experience any undue pain, redness or drainage at an incision site or if you develop a fever.

APPENDECTOMY

The appendix is a small, worm-like structure growing out of the cecum, the beginning of the large intestine in the lower right abdomen. The appendix, which serves no purpose, can become blocked and infected by bacteria. It becomes inflamed and swollen, causing pain and fever.

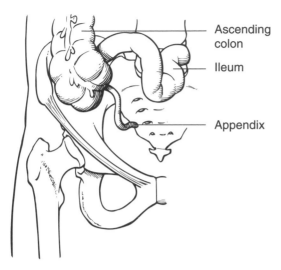

Ascending
colon

Ileum

Appendix

Appendix

If left untreated, the infected appendix can rupture, leading to an acute inflammation of the membrane lining the abdomen (peritonitis). Acute appendicitis is, therefore, a medical emergency requiring urgent attention. Several medical conditions mimic appendicitis, however, and it may be difficult to establish the diagnosis. Certain gynecological conditions in younger women, for example, produce symptoms that are nearly identical to appendicitis.

Laparoscopy is now used to establish the diagnosis in patients suspected of having appendicitis. Most advanced laparoscopy centers also have the capability of removing the appendix with laparoscopic techniques. In cases where the appendix is perforated, patients are sometimes treated initially with antibiotics and appendectomy is performed only after all the infection has subsided. This is referred to as an interval appendectomy.

Before the Operation The diagnosis of appendicitis is usually suspected on the basis of the patient's history, physical examination and laboratory tests. In certain cases, ultrasound is used to establish a diagnosis. Your doctor should inform you that an open operation may be required based on the laparoscopic findings.

Surgical Procedure Laparoscopic appendectomy is usually performed with three small incisions. The laparoscope is inserted through an incision in the navel. A tiny incision is placed on the right side of the belly at the level of the navel and the third incision is made on the left side at the top of the pubic hairline.

If the appendix is found to be acutely inflamed, it is removed with a specially designed surgical stapling device. Because the appendix is infected, it is placed in a small plastic bag before it is passed through the abdominal wall.

After the Operation
◆ After one to two hours in the recovery room, you will be sent to the ward, where you may resume walking and eating within several hours. In some cases, you may be discharged within 24 hours. If there was severe infection, several days in the hospital may be required.
◆ Patients who undergo laparoscopic appendectomy resume their normal activities sooner than those who have a conventional open procedure. The scars are also much less conspicuous than those of open appendectomy.
◆ Non-narcotic pain relievers are usually sufficient to keep you comfortable after surgery.
◆ If you experience any undue pain, redness or drainage at an incision site or if you develop a fever, alert your physician.

QUESTIONS TO
ASK YOUR SURGEON

◆ How long have you been performing laparoscopic surgery?

◆ How many of these procedures have you performed?

◆ Under what circumstances would you convert to an open operation?

◆ How long do your patients stay in the hospital?

◆ When can I expect to resume my normal activities?

9
HERNIAS

F. Charles Brunicardi, MD, FACS

A hernia is an opening in your body that does not belong there. You may notice a lump in your groin that appears and disappears when you strain or cough. When you relax and lie down, the lump sometimes disappears. At this point you should see your doctor. He or she will determine whether you do have a hernia, describe the details to you and discuss the possible treatments.

WHAT CAUSES A HERNIA

Most hernias protrude from the abdomen. The reason for this is that the abdomen contains many internal organs held within the abdominal cavity by the abdominal wall. The abdominal wall is composed of several layers, including a thick, leathery layer made of muscle and connective tissue (fascia). If an opening develops in this leathery layer, the internal organs push out through the hole and create a lump under the skin.

Hernias may occur at any time in your life. You may even be born with one.

◆ People who are born with hernias usually have them fixed as children, but many people don't realize they have a hernia until it has grown over many years.

◆ You may acquire a hernia through any activity that causes damage to the tissues of the body. Heavy lifting or strenuous exercise are the most common activities associated with a hernia.

◆ Certain medical conditions such as chronic coughing or straining with urination or bowel movements may lead to a hernia.

Hernias are a problem, and if you have one, you should have it fixed as soon as possible. It will only get bigger over time, which will make it harder to repair. A hernia may also be dangerous because your internal organs may get trapped in the hole and strangulate. The blood supply to the organ will be cut off and it will eventually die. Strangulation of an internal organ requires an emergency operation with a prolonged hospital admission.

Since the repair of a hernia is usually a straightforward operation, it is preferable to have it done as soon as possible.

PLANNING YOUR HERNIA REPAIR

Most simple hernias are repaired on an outpatient basis. The operation takes about an hour to perform and you can go home after several hours of recovery.

Understanding the Procedure Before the operation, meet with your surgeon to go over all the details, including the potential for complications.

◆ Your surgeon should describe to you what a hernia is so that you understand the concept. There are many types of hernias, and your surgeon should discuss the specific type that you have.

◆ It is important to identify the cause of a hernia, so that it will not come back after it is repaired.

◆ If your hernia was caused by chronic coughing, chronic constipation or straining on urination, discuss how these conditions can be fixed before your surgery.

◆ Your surgeon needs to review the different types of repairs that can be done for your hernia. There are usually several types for each hernia. Each surgeon has her or his favorite repair based upon experience.

◆ Feel free to ask your doctor about her or his experience with hernia repairs.

◆ Ask whether your surgeon will use a plastic patch and about the advantages and disadvantages of this type of repair.

◆ Ask about the possibility of having the repair performed using laparoscopic techniques.

Anesthesia Your surgeon will describe the type of anesthesia to be used and whether you will need to be admitted to the hospital.

◆ Simple hernia repairs are usually done under local or regional (epidural) anesthesia with sedation on an outpatient basis.

◆ Some patients choose to have their hernia repaired under general anesthesia. Many surgeons consider this approach less desirable because the patient cannot cough or strain during the operation to test the repair.

◆ Repairs of complex hernias are almost always done under general anesthesia, and many of these repairs require a hospital admission.

Planning Your Activities During Recovery Ask your surgeon what you can expect during the recovery period, since you may have to modify your daily routine. A smooth, uneventful recovery takes planning.

◆ For example, if you have a job that requires strenuous activity, you must plan to take time off from work, usually about four weeks. You will have to make these arrangements well in advance.

Follow-Up Plan to see your surgeon at least once a few weeks after your repair. He or she will check the wound and review the recovery plan with you.

WHAT TO EXPECT AFTER SURGERY

There are two phases to the recovery period.

First Phase The first phase occurs within the first four days.

◆ In the first few hours after the operation, you will be taken care of by the recovery room staff. You will probably feel groggy from the anesthesia when you wake up and you will feel pain at the incision site. The staff can give you medicine to ease your discomfort.

◆ Your surgeon will describe the plan for pain management after the operation. She or he will give you pain pills to take at home and will discuss their effects beforehand so you know what to expect.

◆ When you are stable, the staff will send you home, accompanied by a family member or a friend. *You should not drive.* The anesthesia will leave you groggy and the quick reflexes often needed behind the wheel can put a strain on the repair.

◆ You will need strong pain medication to control the discomfort on the night of the surgery and the following day, when pain is at its worst. After the first day, the pain usually subsides to a dull ache, and you will require less and less pain medicine.

◆ During the next three to four days,

rest as much as possible and limit your activities to walking short distances. Do not drive during this time. You might want to have your operation on a Thursday or a Friday, so you can rest during the weekend.

◆ If you have a household to run, arrange to have some help, especially if you have young children. You should not be running after children or lifting them up.

Second Phase The second phase of recovery is the one in which the hernia repair will heal and strengthen. This phase occurs from Day 4 through Day 30.

◆ During this time you might experience minor discomfort, but you will be able to resume basic, non-strenuous activities, such as driving and walking longer distances.

◆ You must take great care to protect the hernia repair, so avoid all strenuous activities, such as heavy exercise and heavy lifting, for at least four to six weeks. Otherwise, the repair may be torn apart and the hernia will come back.

◆ People who exercise regularly will have to avoid this activity for at least one month to give the repair a chance to heal. After this period, you will be able to resume your normal activities.

Discuss all these issues with your surgeon, since each will have his or her own advice about your particular situation.

RISKS AND COMPLICATIONS

It is important to recognize what is abnormal after an operation because when you experience something abnormal, it is usually a sign that a complication is occurring.

The most common abnormalities are bleeding and infection, but there may also be excessive pain, a recurrence of the hernia and chronic pain at the site of the repair.

Bleeding, infection and excessive pain are emergencies, so contact your surgeon immediately for these problems. Recurrence of the hernia and chronic pain at the site of the repair are not emergencies, but you should still contact your surgeon as soon as possible.

Bleeding Bleeding complications usually occur within the first 24 hours. A small amount of bleeding that appears as a small stain on your dressing is normal.

◆ With excessive bleeding, either your dressing will become saturated with blood or you will notice a large swelling at the site of the incision. The swelling is caused by blood underneath the skin that is being held in by the sutures.

Infection Wound infections usually begin about four days after an operation. In rare cases they begin sooner.

◆ An infection causes fever, chills, and pain and redness at the site of the incision. The wound will look sunburnt. Occasionally, a reddish fluid or even pus will seep from the wound.

Excessive Pain Some pain is normal after an operation, but it is usually tolerable with pain medication and subsides after a couple of days.

◆ Excessive amounts of pain or pain that gets worse a few days after the operation is a signal that something is wrong.

Recurrence of the Hernia A recurrence of the hernia will usually appear as a new lump at the site of the hernia repair. There can be two reasons for a recurrence: either the repair was performed improperly or the repair breaks down because of weak tissues or strenuous activity. It is very difficult to determine why the hernia has recurred.

◆ If your hernia comes back, contact your surgeon for advice. You may decide to have the repair performed by any surgeon you choose. If your first surgeon does not feel comfortable repairing a recurrent hernia, she or he may refer you to another surgeon.

Chronic Pain The cause of chronic pain at the site of a repair or pain that occurs several months after the operation is difficult to determine. It is usually due to damage to the nerves in the area. This type of complication is very difficult to treat.

The usual steps involve:

◆ observation to see if the pain will subside;

◆ visits to a pain management specialist to see if the source of the pain can be identified and treated with nerve blocking techniques; and

◆ as a last resort, a reoperation to deter-mine if a nerve is trapped in the repair.

If you develop chronic pain at the repair site, have your surgeon thoroughly explain the problem, the plan of treatment and the chances for recovery.

INGUINAL HERNIA

The most common type of hernia occurs in the groin and is called an inguinal hernia. It may appear on the right or left side of the groin.

The groin has weak areas that may lead to the formation of a hernia. There is a naturally occurring small hole in the groin through which the cord to the testicle passes from inside the body into the scrotal sac. If this hole enlarges because of chronic straining or heavy lifting, a hernia—called an indirect inguinal hernia—may result.

Another weak area in the groin is next to the hole through which the testicle passes. This area is called

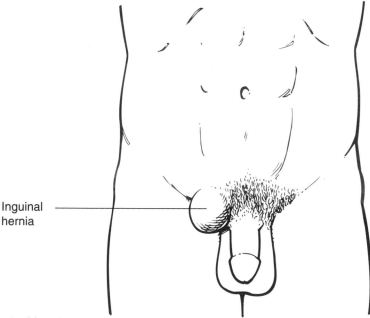

Inguinal hernia

Inguinal hernia

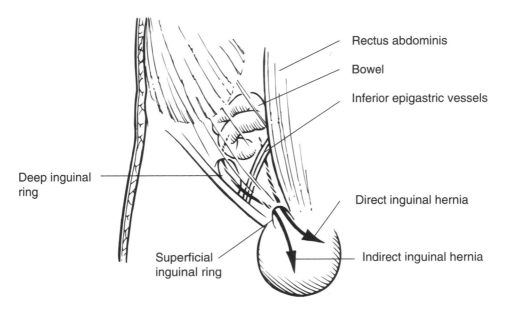

Rectus abdominis

Bowel

Inferior epigastric vessels

Deep inguinal ring

Direct inguinal hernia

Indirect inguinal hernia

Superficial inguinal ring

Indirect and direct inguinal hernias

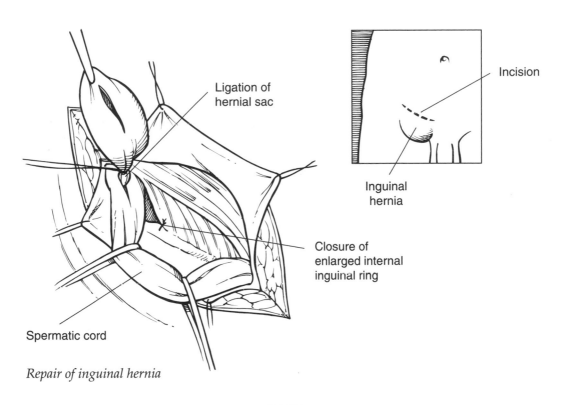

Ligation of hernial sac

Incision

Inguinal hernia

Closure of enlarged internal inguinal ring

Spermatic cord

Repair of inguinal hernia

Hesselbach's triangle. Chronic straining or heavy lifting may cause a blowout of this area, creating a direct inguinal hernia.

The difference between the indirect and direct hernia is like the difference between a rip along the seam of a pair of pants and a tear in the fabric. It is difficult even for surgeons to determine which type of inguinal hernia you have until the operation is performed.

Surgical Procedure Whether the inguinal hernia is direct or indirect, the repair is nearly the same. The repair follows the principles for any hernia repair. First, the internal organs are returned to the inside of the body, which is called reducing the hernia. Second, the hernia sac that held the internal organs is removed. Third, the hole is closed.

There are a number of ways to make the repair. Each surgeon has his or her favorite. You will hear terms such as the Bassini's repair, the Canadian (Shouldice) repair, the McVay repair or the Lichtenstein repair. All these repairs have similarities. The strong tissues surrounding the defect in the groin area are stitched together in a way that the defect will be covered. The repairs differ mainly according to which tissues are used and the exact way the stitches are placed. In the Lichtenstein repair, a piece of strong plastic mesh is added to the repair for additional strength.

Most surgeons repair the hernias from the outside of the body using an incision in the groin, but some are now using laparoscopic techniques to repair the hernia from inside the body. The laparoscopic approach has the disadvantage of being an intra-abdominal procedure. Some surgeons are concerned that this may result in internal scarring, which could lead to future complications. As more experience is gained with this technique, surgeons will learn whether this will be a real problem. Discuss this very thoroughly with your surgeon.

All of the standard approaches result in an excellent hernia repair.

After the Operation Plan on a few days of rest, although you should be able to walk short distances. After several days, you will be able to take longer walks and to drive.

Regardless of the type of repair, avoid heavy lifting and heavy physical exercise for at least a month. Otherwise, the repair may be torn apart and the hernia will come back.

UMBILICAL HERNIA

The umbilical hernia is a common hernia in which there is a hole in the umbilicus (navel). When you strain or cough, the navel becomes larger and puffs out like a small balloon. Usually, you are born with this hernia, but it

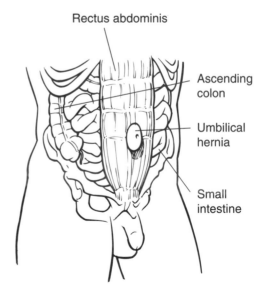

Rectus abdominis

Ascending colon

Umbilical hernia

Small intestine

Umbilical hernia

may not be noticeable until later in life when the hole enlarges.

If your child has an umbilical hernia, your physician will determine whether the hernia should be fixed or just watched over time. Many of these hernias close by the age of four.

Umbilical hernias should be fixed in adults because of the risk of organ strangulation.

Surgical Procedure The principles of the repair are the same as for the inguinal hernia. Umbilical hernia repair is done as an outpatient operation. It may be done under local anesthesia with sedation, although some surgeons prefer to use general anesthesia. As with the inguinal hernia operation, the umbilical hernia repair operation usually takes about an hour. The surgery may be done in several ways.

Many surgeons repair the hernia using a "smile" incision beneath the navel. The internal organs are returned to the inside of the body, the hernia sac is removed and the hole is closed with sutures.

Some surgeons prefer to use a plastic mesh to cover the hole. Once again, each surgeon has her or his favorite way to repair the hernia based upon experience.

After the Operation The postoperative course is similar to that for an inguinal hernia.

VENTRAL HERNIA

This is a hole on the midline of the abdomen. Imagine a line from the bottom of the breastbone to the pubic bone. Any hernia occurring along this line is a ventral hernia.

The same principles as discussed for an umbilical repair apply to the repair of a ventral hernia, although if the ventral hernia is very large, the surgeon

may want to do the operation under general anesthesia and admit you to the hospital for observation.

INCISIONAL HERNIA

This hernia is a hole that occurs in the wound from a previous abdominal surgery. After any operation on the abdomen, the incision is closed in layers using sutures. Most of the time the wound heals without any problem. In rare cases, however, the fascial layer of the wound opens up and a hernia results.

Many people who develop this type of hernia become angry or upset, feeling that the abdominal surgeon made some mistake that caused the hernia to occur. It is difficult to determine the exact cause of an incisional hernia. This type of hernia may occur even when the surgeon has been very careful in closing the incision and everything has been done correctly. Whatever the cause, the hernia should be repaired.

Feel free to return to your surgeon and tell him or her you have a hernia in the incision and discuss possible repairs. Ask how the repair of the incisional hernia will differ from the closure used during the first operation.

If you feel uncomfortable about discussing this with your surgeon or if you feel uncomfortable with his or her answers, feel free to get a second opinion. Some surgeons will feel relieved about your decision to seek another surgeon or may even encourage it, since they may not feel comfortable repairing an incisional hernia.

Surgical Procedure Repairing an incisional hernia is not always a simple procedure. The incision must be reopened, all internal organs must be returned to the inside of the body and the hole has to be closed. If the defect is small, it may be repaired on an outpatient basis.

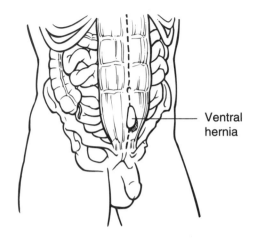

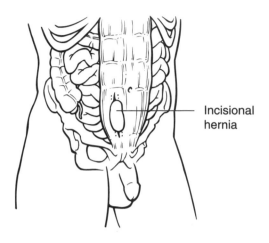

Ventral hernia — Incisional hernia

Ventral hernia

Incisional hernia

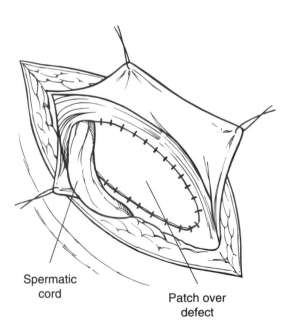

Spermatic cord

Patch over defect

Patch repair

Frequently, the hole is so large that a plastic patch must be used to help cover it. There are other special ways to cover the hole by rearranging the fascial layers of the abdomen. In other words, a patch of your own tissue is used to cover the hole. This usually requires that the surgeon be specially trained in this type of repair.

Most incisional hernias are repaired under general anesthesia. In the case of large and complex hernias, hospital admission may be required. This is because you may not be able to eat right away and may require intravenous fluids and special medications such as antibiotics.

After the Operation Once you go home, you must take great care to protect the repair to prevent a second recurrence.

◆ Avoid any activity such as heavy lifting or strenuous exercise for at least one month.

UNCOMMON HERNIAS

Some types of hernias are so uncommon that even a busy surgeon may have seen them only a few times. If you are told you have one of these hernias, it is important for your surgeon to carefully explain the details about how it might be repaired. Discuss the possibility of having a hernia specialist do the procedure.

Femoral Hernia A femoral hernia occurs in the groin and is found more commonly in women. It is a hole that develops in the space where the blood vessels travel out of the abdominal cavity and into the leg. Usually this hernia appears as a lump at the top of the thigh near the crease in the groin.

A femoral hernia is usually repaired in a manner similar to that of the inguinal hernia. It may also be repaired with an incision in the upper thigh. Both procedures are performed on an outpatient basis.

Spigelian Hernia This rare hernia occurs as a hole in the abdominal wall. A lump is seen under the skin of the abdomen at a point halfway between the navel and the hip bone and can be mistaken for an inguinal hernia. The repair is simple and is done on an outpatient basis.

Lumbar (Petit's) Hernia This hernia occurs in the lower back at the top of the hip bone and is caused by a separation of the back muscles. These muscles form the back wall of the abdominal cavity and help hold the internal organs within the abdomen. The hernia may be first noticed as a lump in the lower back.

When these hernias are found, they should be repaired as soon as possible to avoid the risk of internal organs being strangulated. Whether it is repaired as an outpatient or inpatient procedure depends on the size of the hernia and the person's overall medical condition.

Obturator Hernia This rare hernia develops through a hole in the pelvic bone and may cause intestinal obstruction. It is very hard to diagnose because it occurs deep inside the body and no lump can be felt on the outside. The diagnosis is usually made with a CT scan.

This type of hernia requires a major operation and hospital admission.

DIAPHRAGMATIC HERNIAS

This group of hernias is caused by holes that occur in the diaphragm, the large muscle that separates the abdomen from the chest cavity. These hernias occur deep inside the body and no lumps can be seen on the outside.

There are several types of diaphragmatic hernias that are rare. Some of these are congenital, others occur because of injuries. All the rare types require surgical repair with hospital admission.

Sliding Hiatal Hernia This is the most common diaphragmatic hernia. It occurs where the esophagus, or foodpipe, passes throught the diaphragm to join the stomach. This natural hole in the diaphragm may enlarge and cause the upper part of the stomach to slide into the chest, causing heartburn and indigestion. The diagnosis is made by a special x-ray study called a barium upper gastrointestinal swallow.

There are different ways to treat a hiatal hernia. It is not usually repaired surgically. The symptoms of heartburn and indigestion respond to medical management with antacids or changes in diet. Surgical repair is usually reserved for those patients who have extreme heartburn and indigestion.

Surgical Procedure The surgical repair of a hiatal hernia is an operation in which the stomach is wrapped upon itself to prevent it from sliding up into the chest and to prevent the acid juice from the stomach from being refluxed into the esophagus.

The open operation has always required general anesthesia and hospital admission. Surgeons have now developed laparoscopic techniques to repair this hernia, and it is possible that this procedure may soon be performed on an outpatient basis. Discuss this new type of repair with your surgeon to find out if you would be a candidate for this approach.

QUESTIONS TO ASK YOUR SURGEON

◆ What type of hernia do I have?
◆ How did I get the hernia and how can I prevent a recurrence after the operation?
◆ What types of repairs are there for my hernia?
◆ What type of anesthesia will be needed?
◆ What activities may I do after the repair?
◆ What are the possible complications?
◆ How long will the recovery period be?

10
ARTERIES AND VEINS

Loie Sauer, MD, FACS, *and Jeffrey Pearl*, MD, FACS

—————◇—————

Arteries and veins circulate blood throughout the body. In the process, our cells receive nutrients and oxygen and the waste products of tissues are removed. A constant and efficient blood flow keeps us healthy.

Problems may arise in the circulation system. Arteries may become blocked by cholesterol or be damaged by medical problems such as diabetes, inflammation or trauma. The walls of the arteries may become stretched or swollen (aneurysms). Veins may be blocked by blood clots, become inflamed (phlebitis) or become dilated and inefficient, as is the case with varicose veins. Surgery may be necessary to correct these kinds of problems.

Surgery on the circulatory system is called peripheral vascular surgery. Most of the surgical procedures involved are quite complex and require several days of hospital admission for monitoring and recovery. A few vascular procedures, however, are almost always performed on an outpatient basis. These include treatment for varicose veins, temporal artery biopsies and the implantation of catheters and ports to provide medication, nutritional support or other fluids directly into the circulatory system.

THE CIRCULATORY SYSTEM

To understand all these procedures, it is helpful to know how the circulatory system works.

The heart pumps oxygenated blood outward through the major artery, the aorta, then through a network of ever smaller arteries and capillaries to all the organs and tissues in the body. Veins drain the blood from the tissue cells and return it to the heart. This process is helped by the squeezing action of muscles, especially in the legs, and by valves in the veins that prevent blood from flowing backwards.

PREOPERATIVE TESTS AND EXAMINATIONS

Before considering vascular surgery, your surgeon will perform various tests and examinations to get a clear idea of how your circulatory system is functioning.

Medical History You will be asked questions about any medical history that pertains to the circulation system. Your surgeon will ask about any family history of circulatory problems, any history of blood clots or trauma, about cholesterol levels, high blood pressure, diabetes and whether you smoke.

If you have varicose veins, he or she will ask about your occupation, whether you work standing or sitting, what types of socks or stockings you wear and whether your legs ache or swell at the end of the day.

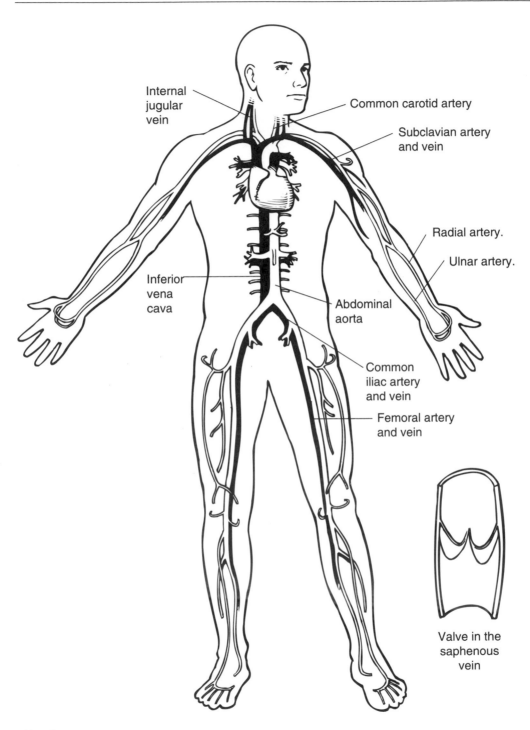

Internal jugular vein

Common carotid artery

Subclavian artery and vein

Radial artery.

Ulnar artery.

Inferior vena cava

Abdominal aorta

Common iliac artery and vein

Femoral artery and vein

Valve in the saphenous vein

Circulatory system

Physical Examination Your surgeon will feel the pulses normally present in the neck, the wrist, the groin area, the top of the foot and the inside of the ankle. A stethoscope will be used to listen to the arteries in the neck and groin.

The veins in the legs will be carefully inspected. You may be asked to stand up or bear down to see if the appearance or behavior of the veins changes with the strain.

Your doctor will note the color and temperature of the skin on your feet and look for any areas of tenderness or discoloration, ulcers or swelling of the ankles.

Non-Invasive Tests Vascular surgeons often want non-invasive tests performed to find out how well your blood is flowing through the system. The information gathered from these tests will be used to clarify your specific vascular problem and help define the treatment options. The information will also be used for comparison after treatment.

These kinds of tests are commonly done in a non-invasive vascular lab, which may be part of your physician's office or may be in a separate facility. The tests may be conducted by your surgeon or by a vascular technician.

◆ A Doppler ultrasound may be used to listen to the veins and arteries to acquire information about blood flow. Several blood pressure cuffs may be applied to your legs so that the leg blood pressure can be measured.

◆ A duplex ultrasound machine may be used to look at the structure of the arteries or veins. The vascular technician will be looking for cholesterol plaques, blood clots or abnormal flow patterns. In the case of varicose veins, she or he will be looking to see if the blood flows backward through the veins instead of forward when you stand or strain.

Invasive Tests Sometimes the surgeon will recommend invasive tests such as an arteriogram or venogram, which provide detailed roadmaps of the blood vessels in areas of concern. These procedures may be performed by a radiologist, cardiologist or a vascular surgeon.

◆ A venogram involves injecting dye through a small catheter inserted into a vein in the foot. The dye shows up on a series of x-rays and indicates blockages or blood clots in the veins. In many cases, it is necessary to obtain a venogram before removing varicose veins to ensure that the deeper veins are functioning normally. In most cases, patients can go home almost immediately after the venogram.

◆ An arteriogram is also an x-ray procedure performed at a hospital, usually on an outpatient basis. The roadmap of the arteries identifies blockages or dilated areas (aneurysms).

ARTERIOGRAMS

Your doctor will advise you about what to eat or drink the day before and the day of the procedure. Fluids are generally encouraged the day before to make sure you are well hydrated, but there may well be factors in your particular case to indicate that fluids should not be taken.

Procedure The procedure is performed in the x-ray department of a hospital, where you lie on a special x-ray table designed to take many pictures in rapid succession. Because the dye used in the procedure can damage the kidneys, an intravenous line will be started to keep your kidneys well hydrated.

Your groin will be shaved and thoroughly cleansed. Large sterile drapes will cover you, leaving your groin open for access by whomever is performing the procedure.

A local anesthesia will be injected into the groin at the site where the doctor feels the pulse in the femoral artery. A needle will be inserted into the artery, followed by a thin wire and finally a small flexible catheter. The catheter will be maneuvered through the circulation system under x-ray guidance until it is positioned at the site to be mapped.

A machine injects dye rapidly while the series of x-rays is taken. In some cases, computer images are recorded instead of using standard x-ray film. You may feel a warm flush inside when the dye is injected, but this lasts only a short time. You will be asked to hold your breath and stay very still while the x-ray images are taken.

After all the x-ray pictures have been taken, the doctor will remove the tube from the groin. Pressure will then be applied on the artery for 20 to 30 minutes to stop the bleeding from the puncture site in the artery.

After the Procedure You will be moved to a recovery room or outpatient hospital room where you will have to lie flat for four to six hours before being sent home.

◆ You will likely be told to minimize your activity for the next 24 hours.

◆ When you are at home, look at the groin every few hours to see if there is any bleeding, bulging or large bruising. Also note any change in color, temperature or sensation in your foot. If any of these changes occur, call your doctor.

◆ Within a few days, you will meet with your surgeon to talk about the findings of the arteriogram and to discuss treatment options. To get a better understanding of the situation, ask your doctor to show you the x-rays.

TEMPORAL ARTERY BIOPSY

A disorder called temporal arteritis, or giant cell arteritis, can produce symptoms such as headaches, visual changes or possibly tenderness in the temporal artery, which is at the temple near the hairline.

Certain blood tests may suggest that you have this condition, and your doctor may refer you to a surgeon for a temporal artery biopsy to confirm the diagnosis.

This is a minor outpatient procedure. It involves removing a segment of the artery so that it can be examined under a microscope to see if the artery is inflamed by a cell known as a giant cell.

Surgical Procedure The biopsy is performed under local anesthesia. Some hair near the temple may be shaved so that the incision is made within the hairline, which will make the scar barely visible when the hair grows back.

The incision may be 1 or 2 in. (2.5 to 5 cm) long. Once the incision is made, the artery is cut, a small segment is removed and the remaining ends of the artery are tied together. This will not reduce the flow of blood to your face because the rich network of arteries detours the blood through many adjacent branches.

The incision is closed with sutures and a bandage may be applied.

After the Operation Complications from this procedure are uncommon, but on rare occasions there may be bleeding, swelling or numbness of the face or weakness in the facial muscles. If any of these occur, contact your surgeon.

◆ The results of the biopsy are usually available within one to three days. If the biopsy shows that you do have temporal arteritis, you may be started on medication to treat the disorder.

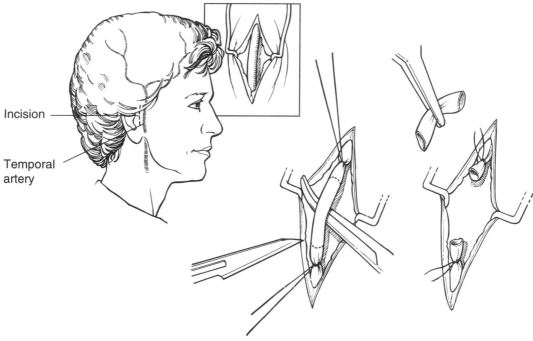

Temporal artery biopsy

VARICOSE VEINS

Varicose veins are a common problem affecting about 10 percent of the adult population in the United States.

Those who have them may suffer from aching legs, swollen ankles, the formation of ulcers, pigmentation and thickening of the skin and the appearance of bulging, bluish veins all over the legs. The appearance is sometimes troublesome to those women who prefer to wear shorts or skirts.

Varicose veins are caused by weakness in the walls of the surface veins in the legs, usually in the long saphenous, or greater saphenous, vein that runs up the inner side of the leg from the ankle to the groin.

Valves inside the veins are supposed to act as trapdoors to keep the blood flowing upwards against gravity toward the heart. But with varicose veins, the valves become defective and weak, allowing blood to flow backward. The veins become stretched and the pressure inside them increases. Much like a plumbing malfunction, the congestion formed by the backup eventually spreads farther and farther away from the site of the main problem. The body compensates for the defective surface veins by making the good deeper veins in the legs work harder.

Surgical treatment depends on the severity of the problem and the size and location of the veins being treated. There are three common methods: injection sclerotherapy, excision of the veins or complete removal (stripping) of the affected veins.

Surgical Procedure: Injection Sclerotherapy This procedure is usually done in a doctor's office. The doctor injects a chemical irritant into the affected veins

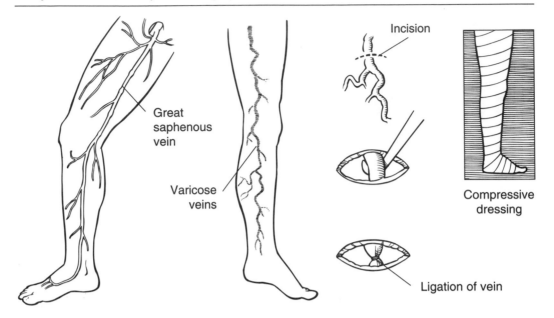

Great saphenous vein   *Vein ligation procedure*

using a very small needle. Each vein is injected separately, so there may be several or many needle punctures.

The fluid produces inflammation inside the vein and makes the walls stick together so that blood no longer flows into that segment of the vein.

After each injection, your leg will be elevated while the doctor applies pressure on the vein. After all the intended veins have been injected, the leg may be wrapped with elastic bandages to minimize swelling.

Surgical Procedure: Vein Excision or Ligation Sometimes minor surgical procedures are used in combination with injection sclerotherapy. These procedures may be done in an outpatient surgical center or in a minor procedure room in your doctor's office.

The entire leg and groin are shaved and cleansed and draped with sterile drapes. Some intravenous sedation may be given and a local anesthetic will be injected into the skin and tissues over

the affected veins. The saphenous vein in the groin may be tied off near the defective valve so blood will no longer flow backward.

Small incisions in the thigh or calf give the surgeon access to some of the dilated clusters of veins, which are pulled out and tied off using an instrument that looks like a crochet hook. Some other veins may be injected the same day or during a follow-up visit in the office. After the procedure, the leg is usually wrapped with elastic bandages to minimize swelling.

Surgical Procedure: Vein Stripping For much larger varicose veins, the entire saphenous vein and the lesser saphenous vein running down the back of the calf have to be removed. This sounds drastic, but as long as the deeper veins are working normally the body adjusts quite well to the removal of the saphenous veins. Preoperative tests will determine whether the deeper veins are functioning properly.

Vein stripping may be done under general anesthesia or local anesthesia with intravenous sedation, depending on the size of the affected veins and whether both legs are involved. The most advanced cases require general anestheia.

The entire leg and groin are prepared and draped with sterile drapes. An incision is made in the groin, and the saphenous vein and several side branches are cut and the ends tied off. Another incision is made over the saphenous vein at the ankle. A plastic tube is inserted into the vein at the ankle and threaded through the vein, up to the opening in the groin. The vein is then cut and tied at the point where it enters the large vein of the leg. The upper end of the vein is now tied to the plastic tube and a cap is placed on the end of the tube so that the vein cannot slide off. The entire saphenous vein is then stripped or pulled out by pulling on the tube. Usually several other incisions are made in the calf and thigh over side clusters of veins that are also removed. The lesser saphenous vein may be stripped from the back of the calf in a similar fashion.

The incisions are closed with sutures, staples or steri-strips, and the leg is elevated and wrapped.

After the Operation You should speak with your doctor about what to expect after each of these treatments.

◆ You will be advised to minimize your activity and keep your leg or legs elevated for the next day or for several days.

◆ Ask how long you should stay off your feet and how long you should wear elastic bandages or leggings.

◆ Injections sometimes produce stinging of the skin and bruising around the vein. Sometimes a lump develops along the path of the vein. Ask your doctor what to do if this occurs.

◆ Some aching and bruising are common after these procedures, and there will be some pain that can be managed by analgesics your doctor will prescribe.

◆ Call your doctor if anything abnormal happens, such as severe pain that isn't eased by the pain medication you've been given, bleeding through the bandages or extreme swelling of the foot or leg.

ACCESSING VEINS AND ARTERIES FOR KIDNEY DIALYSIS

People whose kidneys fail to perform their main function of filtering fluid wastes from the blood have to have their blood purified by an artificial kidney, or hemodialysis machine. The blood is pumped through this machine, filtered, then circulated back into the body.

For anyone who needs long-term dialysis, a connection between an artery and a vein has to be constructed to create a high-flow system that will facilitate access between the circulatory system and the machine.

The connection is usually made in the arm. Once constructed, blood flows rapidly through the conduit. During a dialysis session, needles inserted through the skin into the conduit are connected to the tubing going to and from the machine.

Surgical Procedure The procedure is generally done under a local anesthesia with intravenous sedation. The arm is washed and draped with sterile drapes. An incision may be made over the arterial pulse, either at the wrist or near the elbow crease.

In some cases, the artery may be sewn directly to an adjacent vein. This procedure is sometimes referred to as a Cimino-Brescia fistula. With time, your own veins will increase in size because of

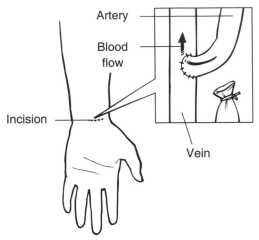

Connection between vein and artery for kidney dialysis

the increased blood flow. The connection to the dialysis machine is made by placing needles into these expanded veins.

Sometimes the veins are not suitable for creating a Cimino-Brescia fistula. In this case, a piece of tubing made of some synthetic material such as Goretex may be tunneled under the skin between the artery and a larger deep vein and then is sewn to each. After a short time, the graft becomes firmly fixed in the tunnel. The tubing from the dialysis machine can be connected directly into the graft. The major disadvantage of this type of fistula is that it is more prone to infection.

Fistulas constructed from your own blood vessels will function for 10 years or more. Most fistulas constructed with synthetic tubing will last only three to five years. Discuss these issues with your doctor beforehand.

After the Operation It is preferable to wait for two weeks or more before using the arm for dialysis access.
◆ Your doctor will assess the degree of swelling in the arm and listen with a stethoscope to assess how well the blood is flowing through the conduit. A

buzzing or vibration along the vein is a signal of a good flow.
◆ Ask your doctor for instructions on how much or how little you may use the arm and hand in the first few days after the operation. Also ask whether you should keep your arm elevated and when you may bathe.

When to Call Your Doctor There may be complications after this procedure, both in the short term and over the long term. Long-term complications may include infection and blockage of the conduit.

Contact your doctor promptly:
◆ if you have any bleeding or profound swelling of your hand;
◆ if your hand changes color or temperature or if there is a change of sensation in your hand;
◆ if you develop pain, redness or streaking in your arm; or
◆ if you can no longer feel a pulse or a buzzing or vibration along the conduit.

ACCESSING VEINS WITH CATHETERS AND PORTS TO DELIVER MEDICATION AND NUTRITION

Treating disease often requires infusing various fluids directly into the circulatory system. Everyone has had a drug injected into an arm, leg or some other part of the body. Many people have had a slow-drip intravenous, or IV, line inserted into an arm for a day or two.

With today's more complex treatments, long-term vascular venous access is becoming much more common. This involves the delivery of medication or other fluids directly into a vein through a small plastic tube, called a catheter, which is placed through the skin.

Many diseases are now treated with

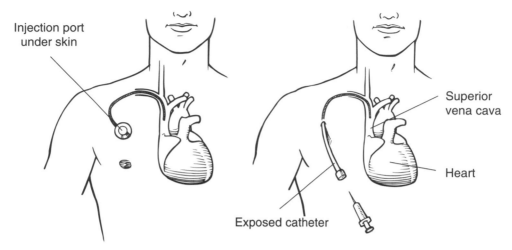

External and internal long-term vascular access

powerful drugs that have to be delivered into the central venous circulation. This requires access to the main large vein, usually the superior vena cava, which drains the blood from the head, neck and arms back into the heart. This is a high-flow, high-volume circuit. Medication delivered into the central venous circulation is immediately diluted, which means it is more easily accepted by the patient.

Long-term access to the central venous circulation is often needed by people with chronic illnesses. After repeated injections, such people finally run out of usable veins. Delivery of medication into the central venous circulation may be their last hope, which is why the catheters are sometimes called lifelines.

Central venous access delivers:
♦ chemotherapy and nutritional support to cancer patients;
♦ nutritional support and multiple antibiotics to AIDS patients;
♦ antibiotics to cystic fibrosis patients; and
♦ nutritional support to people with short bowel syndrome.

Types of Catheters and Systems If your physician decides that you are a candidate for central venous access, there are several types of systems to consider.

With external systems, the end of the catheter is left outside the skin. Medication or other fluids can be injected into the catheter as needed. With an implanted system, the catheter is attached to a small chamber, or port, inserted beneath the skin. Drugs are injected into the chamber with a special needle.

One of the major factors determining which type to use is how long you need a system in place. If you need the access for less than six weeks, a device called an external non-tunneled central venous catheter is all that is necessary.

To lessen the risks of infection in long-term cases, tunneled catheters and implantable systems may be used.

Catheters may be placed in an arm, a leg or in the chest near the shoulder.

Non-Tunneled An external non-tunneled catheter enters the skin and the vein at the same place. There are several types.
♦ The triple lumen catheter has three separate straw-like chambers (lumens) through which fluids flow into the body. This means that various fluids,

such as antibiotics, nutritional formulas or other drugs and supplements, can be given at the same time.
♦ The Hohn non-tunneled catheter has a single lumen.
♦ The PICC (Peripherally Inserted Central Catheter) is a long single-lumen catheter that is usually inserted by a nurse into a vein in the arm at the elbow bend and then is passed all the way up the arm and into the large central veins.

Tunneled A tunneled external catheter travels under the skin for 3 to 5 in. (8 to 12 cm) before it enters the vein. The major advantages of the tunneled catheter system is that it is easy to use and completely eliminates the need for needle sticks. The catheter may be used the day of insertion, it may be used for infusion of all IV solutions and medications, and it is easy to remove.

There are disadvantages, however. Having the end of the catheter outside your body is a constant reminder that you are ill. As well, you will have to take care of the exit site with special bandages. You will have to be careful when bathing and will have to restrict some activities such as swimming.

Although it usually can't be pulled out with an average tug, the external catheter may be dislodged or damaged.

There are several types.
♦ The Hickman is a tunneled external catheter that requires injections of heparin when not in use. Heparin is a drug that prevents blood from clotting inside the catheter.
♦ The Groshong is a tunneled external catheter that has a special valve on the venous end that makes it easier to avoid blood clots. This theoretically means that the catheter doesn't require heparin when not in use.
♦ The Broviac is a Hickman designed for a child.

Implanted An implanted catheter with an attached metal port or reservoir may be used for infusing all IV solutions, medications and products. With the whole system placed under the skin, implanted devices also have the advantage of not requiring you to limit activities such as swimming.

Among the disadvantages of these systems is the need for a needle stick each time the system is used. The port is accessed by inserting a special needle

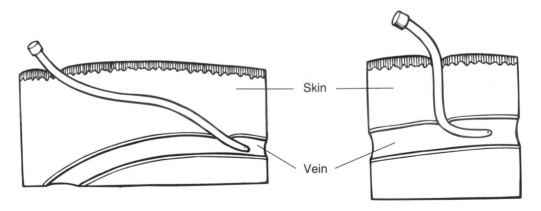

Skin

Vein

Tunneled and non-tunneled catheters

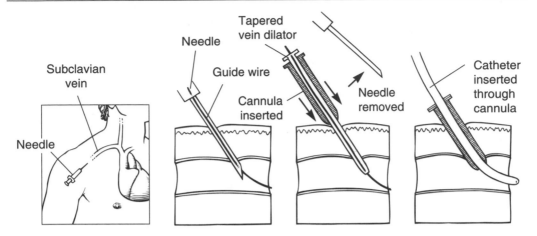

Subclavian vein

Needle

Needle

Guide wire

Tapered vein dilator

Cannula inserted

Needle removed

Catheter inserted through cannula

Inserting catheter into subclavian vein

through the skin and through the port's rubber or plastic cover. Obviously, this is not a good system for people with an aversion to needles. Other disadvantages are that the system can't be used for two or three days after it is inserted and that a small operation is required to remove it.

◆ There are many types of chest ports, which consist of a central catheter and a metal port placed under the skin of the chest wall near the shoulder.

◆ The P.A.S. Port is essentially the same as the chest port but is much smaller and is placed in the arm.

Surgical Procedure All these types of catheters are placed in a similar manner, with the exception of the P.A.S. Port.

In the operating room, your chest will be shaved, if necessary, and your skin cleansed with special soap. An intravenous line will have been started and the anesthesiologist will administer some sedation through the line. You may also be given supplemental oxygen. The surgeon will place sterile drapes around the insertion site, then inject a local anesthetic.

A needle is placed through the skin into either the subclavian or internal jugular vein. A guide wire is then placed through the needle into the heart, with the placement usually confirmed with an x-ray. A dilator and pull-away sheath are then placed over the wire. The dilator and wire are removed and the catheter placed into the pull-away sheath, which is then split.

The catheter is either placed in a tunnel under the skin (subcutaneous), with an exit through the skin at a distant site, or is connected to the subcutaneous port, which is then placed into a pocket below the skin.

The incisions are closed, the position of the catheter is checked with an x-ray, and sterile dressings are applied. The system is then tested to make sure it works properly.

The placement of a P.A.S. Port is done in a small procedure room under local anesthesia. A small incision is made to find a suitable vein (cutdown), and the catheter is fed up to the central circulation. The catheter is designed with a special sensor on the tip so that a sensing device determines the location of the tip. The other end of the catheter is attached to the port, which is then placed into a pocket under the skin 1 in. (2.5 cm) below the elbow crease. Sterile dressings are applied and the system is tested.

After the Operation Discomfort normally lasts only two or three days and is usually taken care of with mild pain pills.

◆ With a tunneled catheter, you will feel some pain at the site of the insertion, over the tunnel itself and at the exit site.

◆ With ports, there will be some discomfort around the implant site.

◆ Generally, these devices won't significantly limit your physical activity. With external devices, however, swimming is difficult, if not impossible, and you must take special care to protect the system when bathing.

RISKS AND COMPLICATIONS

The risks are essentially the same for all central venous access systems.

◆ *Infection*. This is the main risk and a problem with any system. Attention to detail is mandatory when caring for catheters and ports. They require constant surveillance, so it is important that you have a clear and thorough understanding of sterile techniques. Caregivers should explain these to you before you leave your doctor's office or the outpatient surgery center. If a minor infection does develop, it may be treated with antibiotics.

◆ *Collapsed lung (pneumothorax)*. This rare complication (one in 200 cases) may occur when catheters are placed directly into the central veins, which are very close to the lungs. If a lung is accidentally punctured with a needle, air can leak into the chest space and collapse the lung. In some cases, placement of a tube into the chest may be required to reinflate the lung.

◆ *Dislodgment*. The catheter may migrate, slipping in or out of the insertion site. The system may have to be repositioned or replaced.

◆ *Clotting*. A catheter may become clogged by a blood clot. This may sometimes be cleared by instilling a dissolving agent into the catheter.

◆ *Breakage*. Plastic catheters, especially external ones, may crack over time. They can sometimes be repaired with a special kit.

QUESTIONS TO ASK YOUR SURGEON

If you are having vascular surgery:

◆ What exactly is the problem with my circulation?

◆ If my artery is blocked, where is the blockage, what caused it, and is the blockage partial or complete?

◆ Would diet, medication, exercise or time help the blockage, or is surgery necessary?

◆ Would anti-inflammatory medication or support stockings help my varicose veins?

◆ What are the treatment options for my varicose veins and how successful is each procedure likely to be?

◆ How long will I have to stay off my feet after the operation?

If you are having a port or catheter implanted:

◆ What are the differences between the devices that might be implanted?

◆ What kind of anesthesia will be used and what are the side effects?

◆ Will x-rays be used to make sure the catheter is in the right place?

◆ Will there be sutures to remove?

◆ How much pain will there be and how will I manage it?

◆ What are the possible risks and complications of the procedure, both immediate and long term?

◆ If the device has to be removed, how and where will that be done?

◆ What physical limitations will I have?

11
ANUS AND RECTUM

William P. Schecter, MD, FACS

The anorectal area is the final portion of the digestive system. The rectum is the last 5 in. (12 cm) of the colon above the anus. The anus is a 1 in. (2.5 cm) long muscular tube where the rectum opens onto the body surface.

Problems in the anorectum are common and have a wide range of causes, from diet to stress to cancer. Many of these problems may be cured or managed without surgery, but sometimes surgical intervention is necessary.

Several of these surgical procedures are performed on an outpatient basis.

COMMON COMPLAINTS

You may be referred to a surgeon for help with an anorectal problem because you have one of seven common complaints.

Bleeding Any bleeding from the rectum should always be reported to your

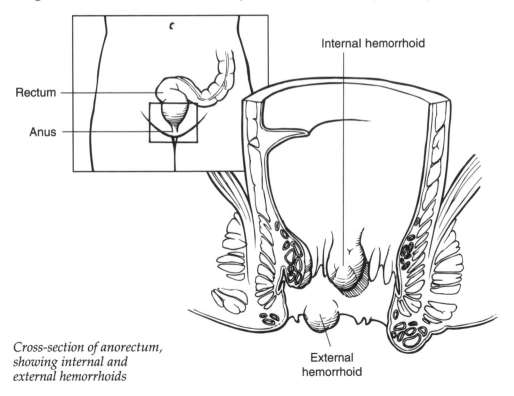

Cross-section of anorectum, showing internal and external hemorrhoids

Rectum

Anus

Internal hemorrhoid

External hemorrhoid

doctor. The bleeding may first be noticed as bright red blood on the toilet paper after a bowel movement. This suggests that the cause of the bleeding is in the rectum or anal canal.

The blood may be noticed in the toilet bowl as dark blood or black tarry material. This suggests that the source of the bleeding is higher up in the intestines or stomach.

Sometimes bleeding may not be apparent at all. Hidden, or occult, blood may be diagnosed by the family doctor with a simple test on a stool specimen. Anyone who has blood in the stool should have further tests to identify the cause.

Pain This is a frequent complaint. Continuous pain or pain associated with a lump is often due to a blood clot in an enlarged vein (thrombosed hemorrhoid). If the pain is worse during a bowel movement, the pain may be due to a split in the lining of the anal canal, called an anal fissure.

Anal Mass The most common cause of a lump or mass in the area around the anus (perianal) is a thrombosed hemorrhoid, but lumps may also be caused by cysts, skin tags or warts (anal condylomata). Occasionally, a perianal lump is caused by a malignant tumor. If the nature of the lump is uncertain, a biopsy should be performed to determine the cause. The biopsy involves removing a piece of the lump or the lump itself for analysis by a pathologist.

Rectal Discharge A discharge of mucus and pus that soils undergarments may be due to an inflammation of the colon, the rectum or the anus. When the discharge is associated with a painful lump, a perianal abscess may be the cause. Sexually transmitted diseases may also cause inflammation of the anorectal area.

Itching Anal itching may be incapacitating at times and embarrassing. There are several possible causes for the itching. It may be related to a rectal discharge. It could also result from an allergic reaction to an undergarment, laundry soap, a lotion or a cream.

Incontinence An inability to control bowel movements may be caused by a variety of conditions, from a disease affecting sensation or muscle function in the anorectal area to a rectal prolapse, a condition in which the rectum protrudes through the anus. Bowel incontinence requires careful medical evaluation.

Change in Bowel Habits New complaints of constipation, a narrowing of the size of the stool or a feeling of incomplete evacuation after a bowel movement raise the question of a growth in the rectal canal. The condition should be investigated.

PREOPERATIVE TESTS AND EXAMINATIONS

When you first see a surgeon about an anorectal complaint, you will undergo a brief general physical examination, which will include a careful examination of the abdomen and anorectum. This will involve a close inspection of the area around the anus, a digital rectal examination and a look at the inside of the rectum and portions of the colon through various endoscopes.

Physical Examination Some surgeons prefer to examine a patient on a special table that allows you to kneel with your chest and abdomen resting on a portion of the table. Or the surgeon may perform the examination while you lie on your side with your knees flexed to your chest.

Your buttocks will be spread and you will be asked to bear down. This lets the surgeon see if there are hemorrhoids or if the lining of the anus and rectum protrudes out through the anus with pressure. A careful search will be made for cracks—called fissures—in the lining of the anal canal. These fissures are often very painful.

The surgeon will then insert a lubricated gloved finger into the anal canal and the rectum and carefully feel for lumps. In men, the prostate gland may also be examined during the digital rectal exam.

Anoscopy In this procedure, a short tube is inserted into the anal canal. The tube is lubricated and its insertion is only slightly uncomfortable. If your main symptom is pain, however, this procedure may be very uncomfortable and the surgeon may choose not to perform this examination in the office for fear of causing you even more discomfort.

As the tube is inserted, you will be asked to bear down. The lining of the anal canal will be carefully inspected. To see the entire anal canal, the instrument has to be turned. The surgeon will warn you before turning the anoscope.

Sigmoidoscopy This procedure lets the surgeon examine both the rectum and the lower portion of the colon. There are two basic types of sigmoidoscope:
◆ The rigid sigmoidoscope is 10 in. (25 cm) long. When it is inserted into the rectum, air is gently pumped into the rectum to inflate it. This allows the wall of the rectum to be examined as the sigmoidoscope is inserted and withdrawn.
◆ The flexible sigmoidoscope is 24 in. (60 cm) long and lets the surgeon examine the entire left side of the colon. Light passes down a flexible fiberoptic cable to the end of the instrument, allowing the surgeon to see the lining of the rectum and colon as the scope is inserted and withdrawn.

Before performing a sigmoidoscopy, the surgeon may ask you to take a laxative or have an enema to allow for a complete examination of the lining of the colon.

Colonoscopy If the main complaint is bleeding from the rectum and the source cannot be found, colonoscopy may be recommended. A colonoscope is a longer flexible endoscope that can pass all the way to the first portion of the right side of the colon (the cecum).

With a colonoscope, the entire colon

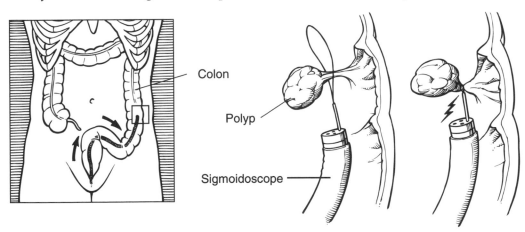

Colon
Polyp
Sigmoidoscope

Colon, showing a polyp being removed with a sigmoidoscope

can be examined. A cleansing of the colon with laxatives is necessary before the examination.

Office Biopsy If a growth is noted in the anal canal, rectum or colon at the time of the visual inspection, the surgeon may recommend that a biopsy be taken. Small biopsies in the rectum are usually quite safe. The main risks are bleeding and perforation of the bowel, which you should discuss with the surgeon if he or she recommends the procedure.

Biopsies are usually performed by a forcep with a small jaw capable of removing a portion of the growth. If the growth is a polyp—a small mushroom-like growth on a stalk protruding into the tunnel (lumen) of the colon or rectum—a loop snare may be placed around the stalk. As the polyp is removed, the stalk is sealed, or coagulated, with an electrical current.

PREPARING FOR ANORECTAL SURGERY

Your surgeon will probably ask you to take an enema both the night before surgery and the morning of the operation. Some surgeons may prescribe laxatives to help evacuate the stool.

Do not eat or drink anything after midnight on the night before the surgery, since having anything in your stomach can result in severe complications while you are anesthetized.

Anesthesia All three types of anesthesia—local, regional and general—are used for outpatient anorectal procedures.
◆ Local anesthesia is appropriate for small office procedures and is achieved with an anesthetic cream or local injection of anesthetic drugs.
◆ Regional anesthesia is commonly used for anorectal surgery.

The goal of regional anesthesia is to anesthetize the nerves in the anorectal area. This is achieved with caudal (local), epidural or spinal anesthesia (*see* Chapter 5).
◆ General anesthesia is an option for major operations or for people who prefer not to be awake during the procedure.

Positioning How you will be positioned in the operating room generally depends on the preference of the surgeon. The surgeon may also consider your height and weight and the location of the problem to be surgically treated.

Anorectal procedures are done in two basic positions.
◆ In the lithotomy position, you lie on your back with your legs suspended in the air and your hips flexed. This gives the surgeon access to the area between the legs and the anorectal region. The lower back area is padded to prevent undue pressure.

The operating team has to position you carefully so that your legs are suspended freely in the air and are not pressing on the poles holding the leg stirrups. If a leg does press on the pole, there is a possibility of a foot weakness developing from pressure on the peroneal nerve, which runs along the side of the leg below the knee. This is a rare problem, but is a known complication of the lithotomy position.
◆ The second popular position is the prone jack-knife position. You lie face down on the operating table, positioned so that your chest and abdomen can move during the breathing cycle. The table is then flexed, giving the surgeon access to the anorectal area.

ANAL FISSURE

An anal fissure is a crack in the lining of the anal canal that may cause severe pain, especially during bowel movements.

The fissure may occur suddenly, be quite superficial and heal with the help of medication to increase the bulk of the stool, frequent sitz baths (soaking the anorectal area in the bathtub or a shallow pan of warm water) and the application of commercially available anorectal creams.

Chronic fissures are deep, long-standing cracks in the lining of the anal canal. Muscle fibers of the internal anal sphincter—the muscle that surrounds the anus and helps control bowel movements—are often seen at the base of the fissure. When you have a painful fissure, this muscle is often in spasm. The pain causes the muscle to contract, which aggravates the healing of the fissure. Chronic anal fissures rarely heal on their own.

Surgical Procedure The treatment of choice for a chronic anal fissure and for an acute fissure that fails to heal after medical therapy is an operation called a lateral internal sphincterotomy. It is performed under local, regional or general anesthesia.

In this operation, the external sphincter muscle is not disturbed. The tight internal sphincter muscle is partially divided. This allows the anus to relax its tone, permitting the fissure to heal. There is often dramatic relief of the pain caused by the fissure after an internal sphincterotomy. Because the internal sphincter is divided laterally, the function of the muscle is preserved and you will be able to maintain control over your bowel movements.

The operation may be done in two ways:
◆ A small incision is made on the side of the anus and the muscle dissected free and partially divided. The advantage of this technique is that the muscle is divided under direct vision. The disadvantage is that to expose the muscle, a 3/4 in. (2 cm) incision must be made.

◆ The second technique involves inserting a thin sharp knife through a small stab incision in the sphincter. The surgeon inserts a finger into the anal canal and feels the division of the muscle. The advantage of this technique is that only a small incision is made. The disadvantage is that the muscle division is felt rather than seen.

After the Operation You will usually be discharged the same day, with instructions to have daily sitz baths and to take stool bulking agents and oral analgesics.
◆ You may expect some degree of drainage for two to three weeks after surgery, and it may be necessary to wear a pad in your undergarments during this time.
◆ The two potential complications to watch for are bleeding and infection.

PERIRECTAL ABSCESS

A perirectal abscess is an undrained collection of pus adjacent to the anus, usually caused by an obstruction of the small glands that drain into the anal canal. The abscess appears as a red, hot, swollen lump that may be very painful. There may be a small amount of drainage associated with the lump.

Surgical Procedure The treatment is incision and drainage of the abscess. Sometimes this procedure is done in the office or a hospital emergency department, but large or extremely painful abscesses usually require general or regional anesthesia to permit drainage.

The operation is straightforward. After the pus is drained, the abscess cavity is packed open with gauze.

After the Operation The day after surgery, the gauze pack is soaked out in a bathtub and you will begin having sitz baths three times a day.

◆ Supplemental antibiotics are not usually required for treating perirectal abscesses unless there is a surrounding soft tissue infection.

◆ The wound may take up to a month to heal.

◆ If the abscess cavity is connected to the anal canal, an anal fistula will develop.

ANAL FISTULA

An anal fistula is a connection between the anal canal and the skin around the anus that causes intermittent pain, swelling and discharge. There is a characteristic nipple-like opening in the external perianal skin, which can sometimes seal over temporarily.

Unfortunately, no treatment short of surgery will cure an anal fistula.

Surgical Procedure The surgeon will examine the anal canal and try to identify the internal opening of the fistula. This is done by passing a probe down the fistula's outside tract. The probe must be passed carefully and without pressure to avoid injuring the tissues and creating a new tract. Once the probe enters the anal canal, the internal opening and the extent of the fistula can be identified.

If the fistula is too narrow for the probe to be inserted, half-strength hydrogen peroxide is injected into the fistula. The bubbles caused by the peroxide may often be seen bubbling through the internal opening.

Once the probe passes from the external to the internal opening, the surgeon cuts into the fistula and opens the

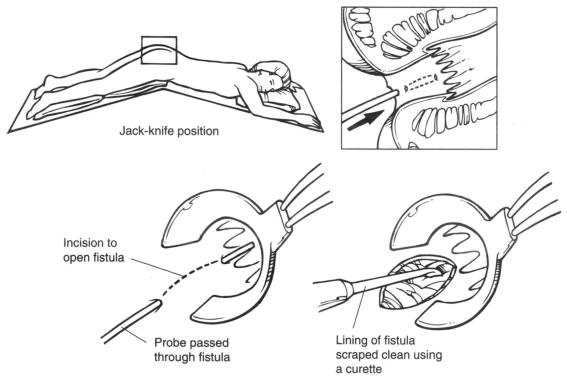

Jack-knife position

Incision to open fistula

Probe passed through fistula

Lining of fistula scraped clean using a curette

Excision of anal fistula

roof of the fistulous canal. The lining of the fistula is scraped clean and the wound packed open.

Occasionally, the surgeon may place a drain (Seton) through the fistulous tract rather than cutting it open. This is done if opening the fistula will result in the division of the external sphincter muscle.

After the Operation The day after the operation, you should begin having sitz baths three times a day.
◆ Healing takes three to four weeks.
◆ There may be a small amount of drainage throughout the healing period.

HEMORRHOIDS

Hemorrhoids are dilated veins in the lining of the anal canal. They may bleed, drop down from the rectum through the anus (prolapse), itch or develop blood clots (thrombose). Thrombosed hemorrhoids are swollen and quite painful.

Treatment depends on the size of the hemorrhoid, the degree of inflammation and the degree of prolapse.

Medical therapy controls the symptoms in most cases. This therapy consists of a high-fiber diet, frequent sitz baths and the use of various commercially available creams or suppositories.

If you have hemorrhoids, avoid straining during a bowel movement and avoid spending prolonged time on the toilet.

Surgical Procedure: Sclerotherapy This is an effective treatment for small hemorrhoids in the anal canal. The surgeon injects a small amount of a chemical irritant into the hemorrhoid to cause inflammation and scar formation that will obliterate the hemorrhoid. This treatment should be limited to small hemorrhoids that do not prolapse.

Surgical Procedure: Rubber Band Ligation This procedure is an option for larger hemorrhoids. It is usually performed in the surgeon's office. A rubber band is placed around the hemorrhoid with the aid of a specially designed applicator. After the loss of its blood supply, the tissue of the hemorrhoid will slowly dissolve and eventually fall

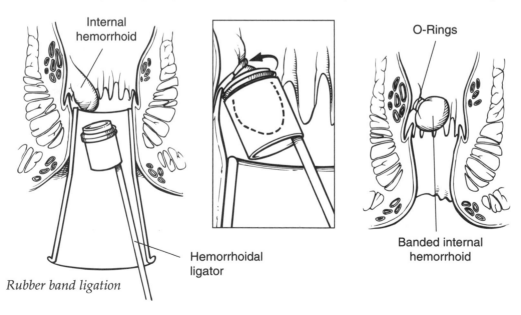

Internal hemorrhoid

O-Rings

Hemorrhoidal ligator

Banded internal hemorrhoid

Rubber band ligation

off. There may be some pain following the procedure and this is usually reduced with sitz baths and analgesics. A small amount of rectal bleeding and discharge may also occur. It is important to avoid taking aspirin, non-steroidal anti-inflammatory drugs and anticoagulants such as Coumadin for at least one week before and for two weeks after the procedure since these drugs may cause increased bleeding.

One of the major concerns of this procedure is the possibility of severe infection, although this is very rare. If you should develop severe pain or a high fever after a banding procedure, return to your doctor or the hospital emergency room immediately to determine whether a serious infection has developed.

Surgical Procedure: Hemorrhoidectomy
Large hemorrhoids that protrude through the anus and don't respond to conservative medical therapy are best treated by cutting them out. This operation, called a hemorrhoidectomy, takes less than an hour and is occasionally performed on an outpatient basis. Most patients spend the night after surgery in the hospital so they can be observed for bleeding.

You will have an enema the night before and the morning of surgery. The procedure is performed under regional or general anesthesia. The positioning of the patient depends on the preference of the surgeon.

After the Operation After any of these procedures, there may be bleeding, thrombosis, pain or infection.
◆ Postoperative care primarily involves sitz baths two to three times a day and the use of stool bulking agents.
◆ Recovery is sometimes complicated by the retention of urine, which may require the placement of a catheter into the bladder.

QUESTIONS TO ASK YOUR SURGEON
◆ How did this condition develop and how can I prevent it from happening again?
◆ What are the treatment options?
◆ What type of anesthesia will be needed?
◆ What are the possible complications?
◆ How long will the recovery period be?

12
EYE SURGERY

David F. Chang, MD, FACS

The eye is particularly well suited for outpatient surgery.

Most eye operations are performed under local anesthesia and last less than an hour. Surgery on the eye has no direct effect on other parts of the body. There is essentially no blood loss, so a transfusion would never be needed. There is usually very little postoperative pain and, since surgery is never performed simultaneously on both eyes, a patient can use the unoperated eye to continue to function normally.

Many eye operations can be performed in an outpatient setting on patients of all ages. Cataract surgery is by far the most common procedure. Other outpatient operations include those for glaucoma, for certain problems of the retina or cornea, for crossed eyes and procedures performed on the eyelids. Laser treatments of eye diseases are performed without incisions and are not considered true "surgery." Nevertheless, the laser equipment is often located in an outpatient surgery center.

THE STRUCTURE OF THE EYE

The eyeball functions like a miniature camera. Light enters through the clear front window of the eye, the cornea, and passes through the pupil, which is the hole in the colored iris.

Immediately behind the pupil is the lens. Just as a camera lens focuses light onto film at the back of a camera, the human lens focuses light onto the retina, at the back of the eye. Like camera film, the retina forms the "picture," which is then relayed to the brain along the optic nerve.

AN OUTPATIENT OVERVIEW

Each procedure performed on the eye has its own set of "normals" in terms of what to expect before, during and after the operation. But there are some standard considerations for most types of eye surgery.

Preoperative Preparations Most eye surgery is not affected by your general state of health, but a brief general physical exam is usually performed.

You will also usually be instructed to continue any medications you regularly take. One exception is anticoagulants such as aspirin or Coumadin. These prevent blood from clotting, so they are often stopped before any operation.

Antibiotic drops to the operative eye are routinely prescribed before surgery to eliminate any germs.

The Day of Surgery Do not wear eye makeup or contact lenses to the outpatient surgery center. Transportation should be arranged, since you will not be able to drive yourself home afterwards. Your ophthalmologist will give

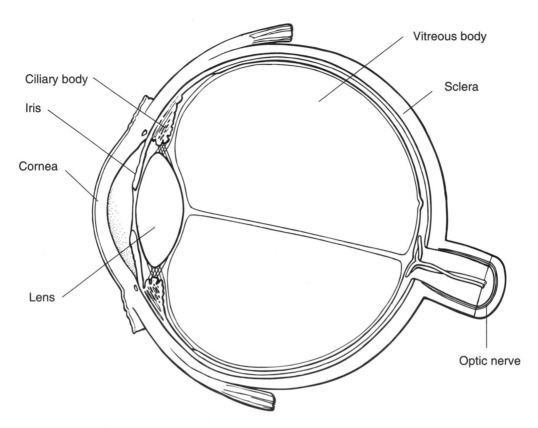

Cross-section of eye

you instructions about whether to eat or drink anything on the day of surgery or to fast for several hours.

At the outpatient surgery center, various drops will be placed in the operative eye. These include dilating drops to enlarge the pupil, which makes the surgery easier. Plenty of time is given to allow the drops to work.

After you change into a hospital gown and lie down on a gurney, an intravenous (IV) line will be started in one arm. This provides the option of giving fluids and medications directly into the vein. Most people are understandably anxious before surgery, so at some point a sedative will be given,

either as a pill or through the IV.

Depending on the preference of the eye surgeon, a device may be used just before surgery to lower the fluid pressure inside the eye. This may take the form of a small weight or a ball that presses lightly against the eyelids. This does not cause any pain or discomfort. Lowering the internal ocular pressure is helpful to the surgeon for many forms of eye surgery.

In the Operating Room After being transferred to the operating room, you will be positioned lying on your back. Once surgery begins, you will be asked to lie very still, so it is important that

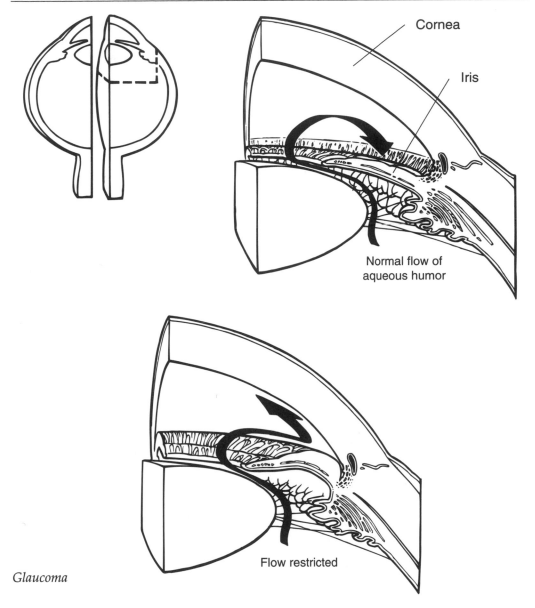

Cornea

Iris

Normal flow of
aqueous humor

Flow restricted

Glaucoma

your neck and back are positioned as comfortably as possible. It is difficult to make adjustments once surgery begins.

As with any other outpatient surgery, routine monitoring of heart rate, blood pressure and respiratory function is performed during the operation. Because your face will be covered with light sterile drapes, a small tube delivering sup-

plemental oxygen will be positioned in front of your nose.

After the local anesthetic is administered, the eye quickly becomes numb. The operative eye does not blink or move, so you do not have to worry about holding the eye still or the eyelids open.

The eye and the surrounding area

are washed with a special antiseptic solution and an adhesive plastic drape covers the eyelids and eyelashes. A small metal device called a speculum is used to gently hold the eyelids open.

During the surgery, you will be asked to close your other eye gently, without squeezing. The surgeon views the eye interior through a special operating microscope, so you may be aware of a bright light shining on the operated eye, but you are not able to see instruments or any details of the operation because the eye is asleep. The eye surface is continually rinsed with saline during surgery, so you may occasionally be aware of fluid running down the side of your face.

Most patients stay awake during the operation. The experience is surprisingly easy because you will be unaware of what is happening to the eye. Mild sedatives may give you a feeling of comfort and relaxation.

You can communicate any needs you may have to the surgeon, but casual conversation is distracting to the operating team and is usually discouraged once the operation begins.

The length of the procedure will vary, depending on the condition of the eye and the surgical method used, but many eye operations are performed in less than an hour.

After surgery is complete, an eye bandage and a small protective metal shield will be placed over the operative eye. You will be taken to a recovery room where the IV will be removed. After having something to drink, you can usually be discharged home right away.

At Home No special care is required at home on the day of surgery. You can eat normal meals and resume any regular pill medications that may have been stopped. Most people spend the first day watching TV with the unoperated eye or napping away the effect of the sedatives. Prescription glasses or contact lenses may be worn if you need them for the unoperated eye.

Depending on the circumstances, you may be instructed not to physically strain yourself or to bend your head forward below your waist.

You might experience a scratchy discomfort if the eyelid doesn't stay shut beneath the bandage, so do not try to open the eye as the local anesthetic wears off. Prolonged reading may become uncomfortable because of the movement of the eye beneath the bandage.

Pain Discomfort after eye surgery is usually minimal. In addition to itching from the bandage, some aching or throbbing of the eye is common as the anesthetic wears off. Reducing your physical activities may help, and regular or extra-strength Tylenol will usually be enough to relieve most postoperative pain. These kinds of pain relievers are preferable to those containing aspirin, which might increase the tendency to bleed.

More intense pain is less common, but should not be cause for alarm on the day of surgery. A stronger painkiller may be prescribed by the ophthalmologist.

CATARACTS

A cataract is a clouding of the normally transparent lens. This causes blurred vision, just as smudges on a camera lens cause blurred pictures.

Most cataracts result from aging and develop gradually. Like gray hair, cataracts are not a disease, nor do they occur at the same age or rate in everyone. Cataracts are the most common cause of blurred vision for people over 50. There is no medicine to cure cataracts, but surgical removal of the cataract and its replacement with a lens implant can restore lost vision for most people.

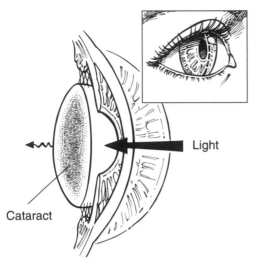

Cross-section of eye, showing cataract

Because cataracts do not harm other parts of the eye, nothing needs to be done until the symptoms of decreased vision are bothersome. As activities such as reading and driving become increasingly affected, surgery becomes a logical option with an excellent prognosis.

Although general anesthesia is an option, most people prefer to have local anesthesia. The eye area can be thoroughly numbed using a local anesthetic to block pain and any movement of the eye or lids during surgery. A long-acting anesthetic is used to lessen postoperative discomfort.

Surgical Procedure Cataract surgery is microsurgery, performed with an operating microscope. It is performed inside the eye through a small incision from either the side or beneath the upper lid.

There is a common misconception that cataracts are removed with lasers. The precision microsurgical tool used to remove the clouded lens is not a laser but an ultrasonic device called a phacoemulsifier. This breaks the cataract up into small particles that are vacuumed away.

To take the place of the clouded lens, a tiny artificial lens is implanted into the eye. This intraocular lens implant is permanent and carries a power specifically calculated for your eye. It cannot be felt and does not change the appearance of the eye.

After the Operation Although the amount of discomfort on the day of surgery varies, pain is not common after the first night.

◆ Your eye will be checked in the ophthalmologist's office the morning after the operation. How well the eye sees when the patch is first removed varies enormously and is not all that important. In most people, vision will be quite blurred or foggy for several days or even weeks.

◆At this visit, the ophthalmologist will check the general condition of the eye and measure the eye fluid pressure. Precautions and instructions will be reviewed and eyedrops will be prescribed. A second follow-up appointment will usually be scheduled for a week or so.

◆ Swelling or minor bruising of the lids may occur and the eye may appear very red at first. These are normal and last about a week or so.

◆ You may get a scratchy feeling in your eye when you blink and eyedrops may burn more than usual.

◆ The eye may water. Secretions that collect on the lids in the morning can be gently washed off with a warm washcloth.

◆ At first, the operated eye will be sensitive to bright light, but this will gradually decrease during the first few weeks. It may be more comfortable to wear dark sunglasses when outdoors, but since the lens implant contains an ultraviolet blocking agent, sunglasses are not needed for medical reasons.

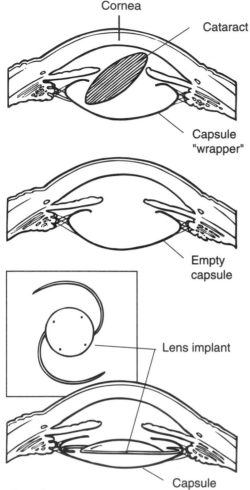

Cornea

Cataract

Capsule
"wrapper"

Empty
capsule

Lens implant

Capsule

*Procedure to remove
cataract and implant new lens*

When to Call Your Ophthalmologist
Some unexpected symptoms should be promptly reported to your ophthalmologist, including severe or unusual pain, excessive discharge or a sudden decrease in vision.

Floaters, which appear as small spots in the line of vision, are often more noticeable after eye surgery, but are not a cause for concern. However, a shower of tiny dots or multiple bright lightning flashes in the operative eye should be reported.

Becoming Active Again How fast the eye recovers physically and how quickly normal vision returns varies from person to person. As with all surgeries, there is a wide range of "normals."

♦ The specific surgical method and the condition of the eye will determine how quickly you will be able to resume normal physical activities. You may be asked to avoid heavy lifting and physical exertion for a few weeks. You may also be advised not to bend your head down below your waist, since the blood rushing to your head will put pressure on the eyeball.

♦ Coughing and sneezing do not cause any problem.

♦ It is important not to rub or press the eye too firmly. You may be given a special metal eye shield to tape over the eye during sleep, which will prevent you from accidentally poking or rubbing the eye. The ophthalmologist will determine how long you have to use the shield.

♦ Soap and water are not harmful, so there is no danger in showering or washing your hair. However, they may irritate some eyes enough for the patient to want to wait a few days before getting the eyes wet. In the meantime, you can wear a shower cap to cover the operated eye. For the same reason, it may be advisable to not wear makeup for a few days.

♦ You can generally resume reading, television watching and normal household activities right away.

♦ You may resume driving or return to work whenever you feel comfortable.

♦ Check with your ophthalmologist about when you may resume exercising, other than walking, or do physical labor.

Recovering Your Vision Many factors affect how quickly your vision recovers, including the surgical method, the health of the rest of the eye and your age and eyeglass prescription. Only your ophthalmologist can give you a realistic estimate of your visual recovery time.

◆ Vision in the operated eye may be very blurry immediately after surgery, but often begins to improve during the first week. Fluctuating vision is common. There is wide variability in the normal recovery rate, even between the two eyes of one patient.

◆ As the eyesight clears, it still may not seem in proper focus until your eyeglass prescription is updated. This is because surgery almost always changes the prescription of the eye. Wearing your original glasses will often increase the blur of the operative eye. This is not harmful, but you may have to adapt because the glasses will still work for the unoperated eye. Initially, you may need to rely on the unoperated eye.

◆ Because the focus of the operated eye usually fluctuates in the beginning, glasses are usually not prescribed until a stable point is reached. This may take from one to three months after surgery. No harm can result from using the operated eye in the meantime for your usual activities such as reading, watching TV or driving.

USING EYEDROPS

Eyedrop medications will be used temporarily to prevent infection and suppress excessive inflammation. This lets the eye heal and become comfortable more quickly.

Your ophthalmologist will determine how often and for how long the various eyedrops should be used, depending on the response of the eye. Any usual eyedrops or medications for your other eye can be continued, as they will not have any effect on the operated eye.

Many patients have their first experience with instilling eyedrops at the time of their eye surgery. The procedure is easy to master with practice and patience. You should note that it is not

unusual for drops to sting, especially after surgery.

◆ Wash your hands. Sit or stand with your head tilted back (some people find it easier to lie down) and look up with both eyes.

◆ Gently pull the lower eyelid down with a finger, creating a "pocket." Invert the bottle and tap it gently so that the drop lands on the eye surface anywhere between the eyelids. Do not touch the bottle tip to the eye or eyelids.

◆ After instilling the drop, close your eyelids gently and keep them closed, without squeezing or blinking, for one to two minutes. This prevents you from blinking the drop out of the eye and through the tear duct into your throat. Passage of drops into the throat is not harmful, but this is why you can sometimes taste the eyedrops.

◆ One drop is adequate, although if you think you've missed, a second drop is not harmful. Some people have trouble telling if the drop landed in the eye, and it may help to refrigerate the bottle, since a cold drop is more easily felt.

◆ If you are using more than one type of eyedrop, wait at least five minutes between using each. Otherwise, the first drop will be washed out by the second.

QUESTIONS TO ASK YOUR OPHTHALMOLOGIST

◆ Are there any other health problems in my eye besides the one you are treating surgically?

◆ What anesthetic do you recommend?

◆ Will I have any restrictions on my activities after the operation? For how long?

◆ When should I have my eyeglass prescription updated?

◆ How long will it take for my vision to recover?

13
EAR, NOSE AND THROAT SURGERY

Jennifer F. Bock, MD, and Mark I. Singer, MD

———————◇———————

Ear, nose and throat surgery (otolaryngology) is a comprehensive surgical specialty that involves medical and surgical treatments.

An ENT surgeon is a highly trained surgical specialist who has completed at least four years of a specialized postgraduate residency program, acquiring extensive knowledge and skills in the management of a variety of ENT disorders. Some ENT surgeons pursue additional training in specialized areas such as head and neck cancer surgery, pediatric ENT surgery, facial plastic surgery and ear surgery.

In the past, people undergoing ENT procedures such as a tonsillectomy stayed in the hospital for several days, but with the advent of short-acting anesthetics and microscopic, endoscopic and laser surgical techniques, it is now possible to perform such procedures as outpatient operations.

Many common problems, including ear infections, tonsillitis, nasal septum deviations, sinusitis and voice (laryngeal) disorders, are treated in outpatient surgery centers.

PREPARING FOR SURGERY

Before your operation, you will meet with your ENT surgeon to discuss the goals and risks of your surgery and what you may expect after the operation.
◆ In some ENT procedures, various instruments have to be placed in your mouth, so at this meeting it is important to tell your surgeon about any loose teeth or dental work that could be damaged by the instruments or by manipulation of the dental structures.
◆ Also inform your ENT surgeon about any drug allergies you have so he or she can select the most appropriate pain medication and, if necessary, the appropriate antibiotic.
◆ If you are taking any medications, ask your surgeon or anesthesiologist whether you should take them on the morning of your operation.

THE STRUCTURES OF THE THROAT

The larynx, or voice box, is a structure in the midline of the neck. It is composed of a series of cartilages and small regulatory muscles.
◆ The thyroid cartilage houses the vocal cords and is particularly prominent in men (the Adam's apple). Vocal quality is modulated by adjusting the tension of the vocal cords.
◆ The larynx is attached above to the epiglottis, a petal-shaped structure connected to the thyroid cartilage. The larynx acts as a trapdoor that prevents the entry of food particles into the windpipe (trachea) while swallowing. The larynx also warms and humidifies outside air on its way to the lungs.
◆ The vocal cords may be likened to the

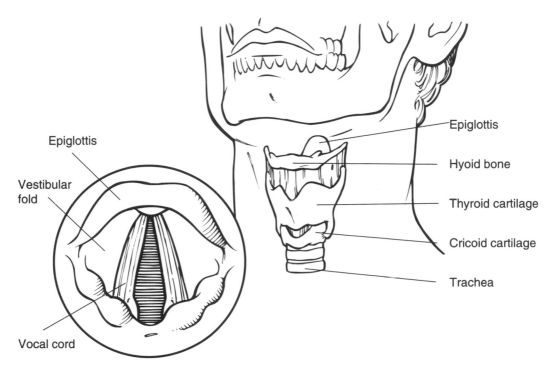

Epiglottis

Vestibular fold

Vocal cord

Epiglottis

Hyoid bone

Thyroid cartilage

Cricoid cartilage

Trachea

Vocal cords as seen from above

Front view of larynx

double reed of an oboe or bassoon. If debris accumulates on the reed or if the shape of the reed is altered by warping, the quality of the sound emitted by the instrument is also altered.

Similarly, if a growth develops on the smooth surface of a vocal cord, air escapes between the vocal cords during speech. The voice then loses its normal crisp quality and starts to sound coarse. If one of the vocal cords is paralyzed and a greater amount of air escapes between the vocal cords, the voice will sound breathy. The quality of the voice may also be changed if one of the vocal cords is stiffened or fixed by a tumor.

LARYNGOSCOPY AND BIOPSIES

Most laryngeal disorders are readily detected in the ENT clinic by looking at the vocal cords while asking the patient to make sounds. Vocal cords are looked at with a laryngeal mirror (indirect laryngoscopy) or with a fiberoptic instrument passed through the nose and down to the level of the vocal cords (fiberoptic laryngoscopy).

To perform laryngeal operations, your surgeon may recommend direct laryngoscopy, which is performed in an operating room, under general anesthesia, with a special instrument called a laryngoscope. This is a stainless steel tube with a light source that allows the operator to closly examine the laryngeal anatomy. With this method, the surgeon can see the vocal cords directly, discover the extent of a disease, take a biopsy and establish a precise tissue diagnosis.

Types of Laryngeal Conditions A variety of throat conditions are diagnosed and treated on an outpatient basis.

◆ Calluses—vocal nodules or singers' nodules—may develop in people who speak frequently or misuse their voice. These nodules usually occur on both vocal cords and produce a hoarse voice. If speech therapy fails to resolve the problem, the nodules may be removed with direct laryngoscopy.

◆ Laryngeal cysts are benign growths caused by entrapment of a mucous gland in the lining of the vocal cord. These generate an abnormal voice and are surgically managed in the same way as vocal nodules.

◆ Laryngeal papillomas are grape-like clusters of tissue that accumulate and proliferate on the laryngeal structures. Papillomas are caused by a virus and should be removed with direct laryngoscopy and laser therapy to prevent them from growing into the trachea and lungs. Unfortunately, papillomas tend to recur, and multiple operations are required to cure the disease. Papillomas are aggressive in very young children and may cause airway problems.

◆ Vocal cord paralysis is often a benign problem. The paralysis may occur spontaneously without an identifiable source, or may result from previous injury, surgery or a tumor. To improve the quality of the voice, Teflon may be injected into the paralyzed vocal cord while you are either awake (indirect laryngoscopy) or under general anesthesia (direct laryngoscopy). The choice of technique depends on the surgeon's preference and your own needs.

◆ Laryngeal cancer usually occurs in people older than 50 and is commonly due to the use of tobacco or alcohol. If your surgeon is concerned about the possibility of cancer, she or he may decide to perform direct laryngoscopy to assess the laryngeal structures and to biopsy any abnormal areas. If malignancy is suspected, your ENT surgeon may pass a scope through your esophagus (esophagoscopy) to rule out an associated tumor in this location.

Surgical Procedure Laryngoscopy procedures are performed under general anesthesia. The reflex that closes the vocal cords is the last activity to be diminished with general anesthesia, and it is very important to have complete relaxation of the protected larynx.

In the operating room, your airway will be secured with an endotracheal tube. Anesthetic gases and oxygen will be delivered through this tube during the procedure.

The surgeon will place a special dental guard over your upper teeth to protect them from injury by the laryngoscope. Your surgeon may also use an operating microscope to get a closer look at any abnormal structures and to guide his or her maneuvers.

The vocal cords are delicate structures. To minimize surgical injury, a carbon dioxide laser may be used to vaporize a benign growth. Occasionally, small malignancies are also treated this way, although most laryngeal cancers require further surgery and/or radiation to remove the tumor completely.

After the Operation You may temporarily notice blood-streaked saliva and have some discomfort at a biopsy site.

◆ Laryngeal and muscular pain may result from the paralyzing agents used in general anesthesia. These problems usually clear up within 48 hours.

◆ Most people resume their regular diet and activities 24 hours after surgery.

◆ If you also underwent an examination of the esophagus with a scope, alert your surgeon immediately if you experience back pain or develop a fever. These symptoms may indicate an injury to the esophagus.

THE MIDDLE EAR

The ear drum, or tympanic membrane, is a tent-like structure draped over the three bones of the middle ear, the incus, malleus and stapes. (Because of their shapes, these bones are sometimes called the anvil, hammer and stirrup.) It is through these structures that sound is conducted to the brain.

Behind the tympanic membrane lies a space, the middle ear space, which is ventilated by the eustachian tube. This tube connects the middle ear space to the region behind the nose, the nasopharynx, where the adenoid tissue is found. Adenoids are lymph tissues above and behind the palate, which may block the eustachian tube.

Obstruction of the eustachian tube produces negative pressure in the middle ear space, which favors the accumulation of pus. If the pressure is too great, the tympanic membrane will rupture, causing a mild to moderate hearing loss and an ear that may become chronically infected.

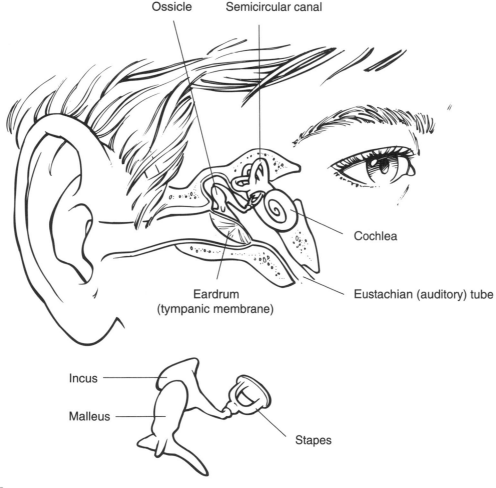

Ossicle   Semicircular canal

Cochlea

Eardrum
(tympanic membrane)

Eustachian (auditory) tube

Incus

Malleus

Stapes

Ear

MIDDLE EAR INFECTIONS

People who have frequent middle ear infections usually complain of hearing loss and severe ear pain.

Most infections clear up with antibiotics, but chronic ear infections develop in some individuals whose eustachian tubes function poorly or who have large adenoids. Adenoids are smaller and much less prominent in adults, so this problem is prevalent in young children.

Surgical Procedure To avoid these problems, a tube is placed through the tympanic membrane into the middle ear space to serve the function of the eustachian tube (myringotomy). This procedure is performed under local anesthesia or, for children, with mask anesthesia.

After the Operation There may be some discomfort from the procedure, but this usually goes away within 48 hours.
◆ You may note some short-term bloody discharge from the operated ear.
◆ As long as the tube is in position, it is important to prevent infections by preventing the entry of water into the middle ear space. If you have tubes, do not swim in unchlorinated water. Before bathing, place cotton with Vaseline in the ear canal.
◆ On average, the myringotomy tube remains in position for six months and then will fall out spontaneously. The small perforation in the tympanic membrane usually heals on its own.

RUPTURED EAR DRUMS

Perforations in the tympanic membrane that do not heal by themselves are closed in an operation called a tympanoplasty.

Surgical Procedure The tympanoplasty is performed under general or local anesthesia and involves patching the rupture by grafting tissue to the edges of the perforation. The ear canal is then filled with a surgical packing to allow the graft to heal.

After the Operation Your surgeon will ask you to keep the ear dry until the packing is removed in one or two weeks. She or he may also suggest applying antibiotic ear drops.
◆ Your surgeon will ask you to avoid flying and scuba diving until the ear drum is healed.
◆ While the packing is in place, you will notice that your hearing is muffled. This is normal.
◆ To prevent the graft from dislodging, avoid blowing your nose with your mouth closed and sneezing with your mouth closed.
◆ Report any infections, bleeding or fever to your ENT surgeon.

MIDDLE EAR RECONSTRUCTION

In genetically predisposed people, the bones of the middle ear may become fused with excess calcium deposits (otosclerosis). The chain of middle ear bones then loses its mobility, resulting in hearing loss. The middle ear bones may also become separated in a head injury.

In both cases, the bones of the middle ear have to be reconstructed (ossicular reconstruction). The procedures, which may involve removing bones such as the stapes (stapedectomy), are routinely performed in an outpatient surgery center.

Surgical Procedure The tympanic membrane is cut and lifted up. The fixed bones are removed and the mobility of the bony chain is restored with an artificial stapes.

After the Operation Postoperative care is essentially the same as for tympanoplasty. Keeping the ear canal dry until the packing is removed is essential.

◆ Pain and bleeding should clear up within 48 hours.

◆ If you develop severe dizziness, facial paralysis or infection, inform your surgeon immediately.

TONSILLECTOMY

The lymph tissues in the back of the throat (the tonsils) and behind the palate (the adenoids) make up an area known as Waldeyer's ring.

In children and some adults, these tissues may become enlarged and chronically infected. When the tonsils are repeatedly inflamed (tonsillitis), their removal is necessary. This procedure, called a tonsillectomy, is also required if your doctor suspects a tonsillar cancer.

A tonsillectomy may be performed in conjunction with an operation for snoring called a uvulopalatopharyngoplasty (UPPP). This procedure reduces some of the excessive soft tissue in the back of the throat to eliminate snoring and

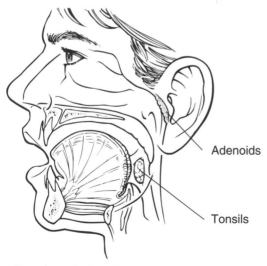

Tonsils and adenoids

sleep apnea, a breathing disorder that occurs when these tissues relax during deep sleep. A portion of the soft palate and the tonsils are removed.

Surgical Procedure Tonsillectomy is a common outpatient procedure and is usually performed under general anesthesia. The ENT surgeon will place a special gag in your mouth to keep the tongue away from the operating area. The tonsils will be cut away. Open, bleeding vessels will be sealed with an electrical heating device called a cautery.

If you are also undergoing a UPPP, the soft palate is trimmed and sutures are placed to tighten the muscles in the back of the throat.

After the Operation After surgery, your tongue may be mildly swollen and numb. This is normal.

◆ Your throat will be very sore for one or two weeks. Pain is the most common complaint after a tonsillectomy, but it is controlled with oral painkillers. Aspirin and non-steroidal anti-inflammatory medications may cause bleeding, so they should be avoided.

◆ You will need to drink plenty of fluids to prevent dehydration.

◆ If you have had a UPPP, your nose will feel blocked for a week or two. This is an expected sensation and will go away as the soft palate swelling diminishes.

REMOVING ADENOIDS

Children who have recurrent ear infections despite multiple antibiotics and despite having a set of ventilating tubes implanted in their ears will benefit from an adenoidectomy. This involves removing the lymph tissue that is blocking the eustachian tube.

The removal of adenoid tissue in an adult is usually done only to rule out the possibility of tumor.

Adenoidectomy is often done in conjunction with a tonsillectomy.

Surgical Procedure The surgeon will place a gag in your mouth and slip rubber tubes into your nose to elevate the soft palate. The surgeon uses a mirror to examine the nasopharynx and removes the adenoids with a special curved blade.

After the Operation As with the tonsillectomy, your throat will be very sore for a week or two.
◆ Any episodes of bleeding should be reported immediately to your otolaryngologist.
◆ Maintaining hydration after surgery is important. Drink plenty of fluids and stick to a soft diet for the first week after the operation.

DEVIATED NASAL SEPTUM

The nose is made up of a series of cartilage and bony structures that give the nose its shape and permit the free passage of air into the lungs. The nasal septum is a piece of cartilage separating the right side of the nose from the left.

Some people are born with a curved septum (deviated nasal septum) that blocks one or both sides of the nose and contributes to "mouth breathing." A deviated septum may also result from a nasal fracture caused by an accident or a fight.

Surgical Procedure To repair a deviated nasal septum, your ENT surgeon will perform an operation called a septoplasty. This is performed under general or local anesthesia.

The operation involves making incisions along the septum to remove bent portions of cartilage and/or bone. External parts of the nose are not removed.

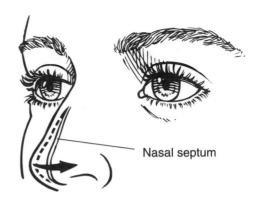

Deviated septum

Packing is placed inside your nose to control bleeding. Sometimes, plastic splints are sutured to the septum to lend additional support during healing.

After the Operation Your nose will be tender inside, but you will not have any external swelling or bruising.
◆ The packing is usually removed a day or two after surgery.
◆ Plastic splints are removed one to two weeks later, in the clinic.
◆ It is not uncommon to have pain and nasal congestion for one to two weeks after surgery.
◆ Small amounts of postoperative bleeding are normal, but persistent, copious bleeding should be reported to your otolaryngologist.
◆ Alert your surgeon immediately if you develop a fever, a rash or diarrhea while the packing is in place.

SINUSITIS

The sinuses are bony pockets within the skull that drain into the nose. There are four sets of sinuses: the frontal, ethmoid, maxillary and sphenoid.

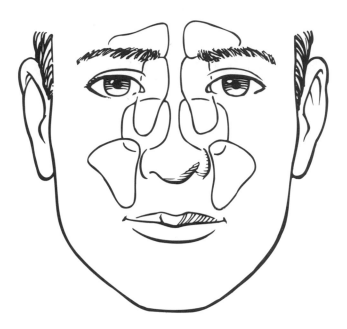

Sinuses and nasal anatomy

The sinuses may become infected if the natural drainage routes are blocked (sinusitis). Sinusitis causes headaches and pain within or between the eyes. The condition is treated with sinus medication or antibiotics, but surgery to drain the sinuses may be necessary after multiple bouts of sinusitis.

Surgical Procedure The goal of sinus surgery is to re-establish the normal drainage flow of the sinuses by opening the bony portals with specialized instruments (endoscopic sinus surgery). This procedure is done under general or local anesthesia.

Narrow tubes with a fiberoptic light source are passed into the nose to examine the nasal anatomy. The areas of obstruction are identified and reopened. If pus is encountered, a specimen is collected for laboratory analysis.

Packing is placed into the nasal cavity to reduce bleeding.

After the Operation The postoperative course and potential complications are much the same as for nasal septal surgery, but with sinus procedures you may notice external bruising.

◆ After surgery, your otolaryngologist will remove the nasal packing in the office and may suggest a nasal irrigation routine to reduce crusting and speed healing.

◆ If you develop severe headaches, neck stiffness or any visual changes, notify your surgeon immediately.

QUESTIONS TO ASK YOUR ENT SURGEON

◆ What is your training, and what is your experience with the procedure I will be having?

◆ How long will my period of disability last?

◆ When will I be able to get back to my normal activities?

14
PLASTIC AND RECONSTRUCTIVE SURGERY

Issa Eshima, MD

With the spread of outpatient surgery centers, costs for plastic, or cosmetic, surgery have been driven down to a point where many more people can now afford such procedures. As well, more people are interested in having cosmetic surgery, which reflects a greater interest in health and longevity.

Plastic surgery and what it represents is often distorted or exaggerated in the popular media, but in the proper context, cosmetic surgery for the well-informed and determined patient is a self-affirming event.

With modern technology, many plastic surgery procedures are performed safely, comfortably and efficiently on an outpatient basis, with local anesthesia and intravenous sedation or with general anesthesia. The advantages include cost savings, a more personal and intimate environment and a more time-efficient system.

DECIDING TO HAVE COSMETIC SURGERY

When you consult a plastic surgeon, you should be motivated yet realistic. The most important question to ask yourself before the consultation is, "What do I want done and why?" There are several issues that have to be carefully considered.

Timing Plastic surgeons often see people who want cosmetic surgery because they recently suffered a divorce, a death in the family, a job loss or some other traumatic event. It is important to understand that a cosmetic procedure is not a panacea. It should not be viewed as a cure-all for life's problems. Patients with such unrealistic expectations are invariably dissatisfied with the result.

There is a time, however, when someone who has suffered a traumatic event has recuperated sufficiently to consider cosmetic surgery in its proper context. This timing is generally determined by the patient, his or her friends and significant others and the cosmetic surgeon.

It is in consultation with the surgeon that issues can be addressed and a well-thought-out plan can be devised. An experienced, well-qualified and well-trained cosmetic surgeon can accurately assess all variables and make a sound recommendation about the timing of surgery, the type of procedure and the potential for success.

Finding the Right Plastic Surgeon
Many people approach a particular plastic surgeon on the recommendation of a friend who has had a similar operation. Often, a family physician makes the referral because of a surgeon's reputation. Then again, you may have to start your search from scratch.

Make sure that the surgeon you approach is formally trained in cosmetic surgery. This may seem self-evident, but many medical specialists do perform cosmetic operations. Some ophthalmologists, for example, who have trained in ocular plastics will do cosmetic eyelid surgery. Dermatologists may perform liposuction. ENT surgeons are trained to perform cosmetic procedures on the head and neck.

Plastic surgeons are required to complete a certain number of years of surgical training before becoming Board-eligible or Board-certified in plastic surgery. Call the American Board of Plastic Surgery to find out whether a particular plastic surgeon is Board-eligible or Board-certified.

A surgeon who has trained in a plastic surgery residency or fellowship typically has expertise in both cosmetic and reconstructive surgery. Reconstructive surgery includes hand surgery, the reconstruction of tissues lost through burns, cancer operations or other causes, and trauma surgery. Most plastic surgeons do a combination of cosmetic and reconstructive surgery, but some perform only one type. This can be determined by a phone call or at your consultation.

During your consultation, ask to see preoperative and postoperative photographs of patients who have undergone the procedure you are interested in. Look at these pictures carefully. Photos can be misleading. The aesthetic improvements may be due to a new hairstyle, weight loss, makeup or better lighting as well as to the plastic surgery.

The surgeon should detail the specifics of the operation and answer all your questions thoroughly. (It helps to take a list of questions with you.) It is most important that you feel comfortable with the surgeon and with the procedure before deciding to proceed.

Smoking increases the risk of skin sloughing and poor wound healing, so anyone having cosmetic surgery has to stop smoking for two weeks before and two weeks after the operation.

Costs Cosmetic surgery is purely an elective procedure. It is not truly necessary, so most medical insurance does not cover the expense. You are responsible for all costs, so you have to assess realistically what you can afford. This can be done in consultation with the plastic surgeon's office. In certain practices, financing is possible.

ANESTHESIA AND SEDATION

Many medications are used to provide adequate sedation and anesthesia during plastic surgery.

◆ If local anesthesia is insufficient, intravenous (IV) sedation may be added or a regional or general anesthetic may be given. With regional or general anesthesia, either a nurse anesthetist or an anesthesiologist will be with you in the operating room.

◆ Throughout the procedure, you will be monitored with several devices. The EKG measures your heart rhythm. A blood pressure monitor with a cuff around an arm or leg measures your blood pressure. A pulse oximeter placed on a finger, toe or earlobe constantly monitors the amount of oxygen in your blood.

FACELIFT

The facelift operation, or rhytidectomy, was first described in medical literature in the early 1900s. The earliest procedures removed wrinkles and excess skin by simply cutting the excess skin away and stitching the wound together. Variations of such techniques evolved into the facelift procedure we know today.

The facelift addresses problems of the jowl area and the sagging neck. It can accentuate the cheek and jawline and remove muscular bands and neck

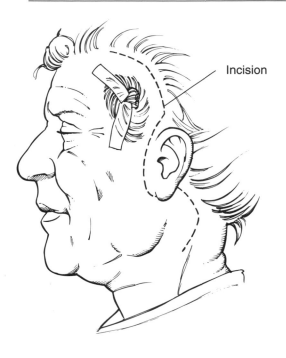
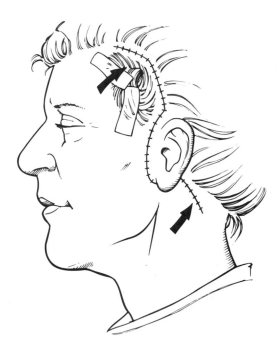

Incision

Facelift

wrinkles. Combined with the removal of fat in the neck (suction lipectomy), the procedure is particularly successful in recontouring the characteristic features of an aging face and neck. It is also quite common to have eyelid surgery (blepharoplasty) at the same time.

The nasal labial folds—the prominent line between the cheek and the upper lip—are particularly difficult to modify, but some newer techniques address the problem with reasonable results.

Surgical Procedure The facelift essentially involves an incision in front of and behind the ear. The surgeon elevates the facial skin and the deeper layers of tissue in such a way as to stretch and rotate the skin of the face and neck. This redrapes the soft tissues of the face over the bony facial structure, producing a more youthful appearance.

Another incision behind the chin, in what is called the submental region, is

often made so that the surgeon can remove the fat and sometimes the muscle bands that are prominent in some people. This incision is usually placed within or near a crease in such a way that the healed incision is barely noticeable.

It is not uncommon for a plastic surgeon to use staples to close the skin in the hair-bearing sections of the face and scalp, but sutures are used to close incisions made in the hairline and in front of and behind the ear. All the stitches are usually removed within 14 days of the operation.

The incision used in the facelift technique involves just the skin or the deeper tissue layers of the face. There are proponents of every technique, so discuss the options with your surgeon. It has been reported that involving the deeper structures tends to produce a longer-lasting result, but this is debatable. How long the facelift lasts depends on the individual.

A facelift takes anywhere from an hour and a half to six hours to complete, depending on the amount of lift needed. You may have drains placed under the skin, which are not uncomfortable and are usually removed the next day.

After the Operation The effects of the operation and the rate of healing depend on both the individual and the extent of the procedure.

◆ Swelling is to be expected for at least a week.

◆ You will usually be instructed to place cold compresses on your face, neck and eyes for 48 hours after the operation.

◆ A soft diet is recommended for the first few days.

◆ You will usually be instructed to move your face and neck as little as possible during the first few days.

◆ Most of the swelling is gone within a week to 10 days, but the optimal result is usually noted one to two months after the operation.

Complications Complications are rare. Rates of 1 to 4 percent are commonly quoted for complications such as:

◆ bleeding or a collection of blood under the skin (hematoma);

◆ asymmetry;

◆ widened scars;

◆ thinning hair (alopecia);

◆ skin sloughing;

◆ infection; and

◆ injury to sensory and facial nerves.

EYELID SURGERY

Surgery on the eyelids, or blepharoplasty, is a common procedure performed mainly to restore a more youthful-looking eye by removing the excess skin and fat that develop naturally with age.

It is also performed to correct a

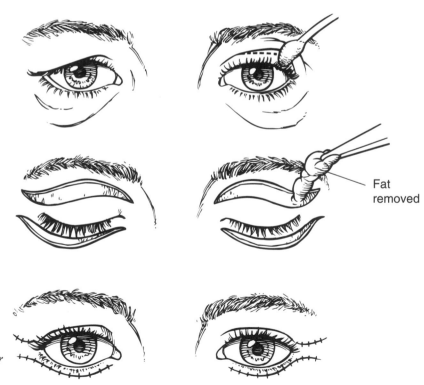

Fat removed

Upper and lower blepharoplasty

condition called dermatochalasia, in which the excess skin of the upper eyelid droops severely. In the most severe cases, this upper eyelid skin obstructs vision.

Surgery on the upper and lower lids typically takes one to two hours, depending on the approach, and is done under local anesthesia, often combined with IV or oral sedation.

Surgical Procedure: Upper Blepharoplasty As we age, the upper eyelid skin, which is extremely thin, tends to become excessive. The fold in the upper eyelid—the supratarsal fold that accentuates the eye aesthetically—can be lost as a result of overhanging excess skin. Fatty pockets accumulate. There are commonly two such pockets in the upper eyelid: the medial and central fat pads. These fat pockets magnify the effect of the excess skin, producing a puffier, more tired look.

The upper blepharoplasty restores the fold in the upper eyelid and removes the fat. The incision is made along the line of the natural fold. After the excess skin and some of the muscle beneath it are cut away and the fat is removed, the incision is closed with sutures, leaving a scar that is barely visible.
◆ Blepharoplasty may involve creating a fold on the upper eyelid. People of Asian ancestry often do not have a supratarsal fold or may have a fold on only one eye. A fold is created by a procedure called a double lid operation, which is frequently performed in Asia today. Care is taken to place this fold 6 to 8 mm from the cilliary line to maintain ethnicity. A higher fold of 10 to 11 mm above the cilliary line is typical of the Caucasian eyelid, and produces an Occidental look in the Oriental face.

Surgical Procedure: Lower Blepharoplasty Usually three fatty pockets accumulate in each lower eyelid: a medial, a central and a lateral fat pad. As with the upper blepharoplasty, these fat pads can be removed and the contour of the eyelid changed in such a way as to make the eye look less puffy and more rested.

The lower blepharoplasty is performed in two ways.
◆ In a subcilliary lower blepharoplasty, an incision is made just below the lashline on the lower eyelid. The advantage of the subcilliary incision is that skin and sagging muscle are trimmed at the same time as the excess fat is removed.
◆ In a transconjunctival lower blepharoplasty, a small incision is made within the lining, or conjunctiva, of the lower eyelid. The advantage of the transconjunctival approach is that fat is removed without a visible scar. This approach is most suitable for people who do not need to have excess skin cut away.

After the Operation With either the upper or lower blepharoplasty, bruising is expected for at least one week and sometimes for up to a month.
◆ Swelling of the eyelids may last until a day or two after any sutures are removed.

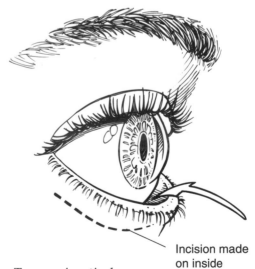

Incision made on inside

Transconjunctival lower blepharoplasty

◆ Avoid strenuous activities for the first two weeks, although you may return to your job after one week depending on the nature of your work and the advice of your plastic surgeon.

◆ Contact lenses may be uncomfortable for a time. Discuss with your surgeon when you may safely resume wearing contacts.

◆ The more severe complications of blepharoplasty include prolonged swelling, asymmetry, infection, bleeding, dry eye and bowing of the lower eyelid (ectropion), although these complications are uncommon.

◆ Blindness has been reported, but this is extremely rare.

BROW LIFT

Brow ptosis is a deformity in which the eyebrow and its accompanying skin drop below the brow ridge because of lax muscles and softening tissues. Brow ptosis accentuates the excess skin of the upper eyelid, a problem that is seen in middle age. The drooping may be more prominent on one side. Correcting brow ptosis requires a brow lift.

The brow lift essentially elevates the eyebrow back to its more youthful loca-

tion and corrects some of the excess skin deformity in the upper eyelid area. In older people, a combined brow lift and blepharoplasty is necessary to correct the entire deformity.

Surgical Procedure A brow lift involves an incision right above the eyebrow, at the hairline or behind the hairline. The type of incision depends on the amount of hair you have, the severity of the ptosis, the proportions of your forehead and hairline and your own preferences.

Most people prefer an incision hidden in the hairline. This incision is called a bicoronal incision and is usually made 2 1/2 in. (6 cm) behind the hairline.

◆ After the incision is made, the entire skin of the forehead is elevated and separated from the underlying tissues all the way to the eyebrows. Various muscles are surgically altered to correct forehead wrinkles and correct the brow ptosis.

◆ This procedure usually takes one to two hours and is easily performed under local anesthesia with IV sedation.

◆ In very select patients, upper eyelid fat may also be removed by this brow lift approach.

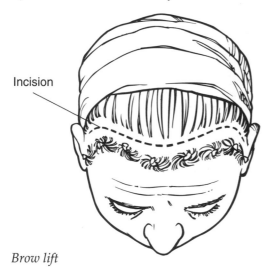
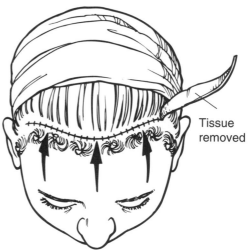

Incision

Tissue removed

Brow lift

SURGERY ON THE NOSE

Nasal surgery, or rhinoplasty, involves contouring the nasal bones and/or reshaping the tip of the nose. Most of these procedures are performed with small incisions inside the nose so that no scars are visible.

Rhinoplasty is also performed for people who have obstructed airways. Typically, these people have a deviated septum because of either a developmental problem or an injury to the nose. Correcting the deviated septum assists breathing, so this procedure is often covered by medical insurance.

Surgical Procedure Rhinoplasty involving recontouring of the nasal bones and cartilage usually reduces the width of the nose and eliminates any hump on the bridge of the nose. The subtleties of the rhinoplasty involve recontouring the tip of the nose and, in some cases, the flare of the nostrils.

For people who have had their noses broken, rhinoplasties involve bracing the nasal bones back in their correct position either by reducing the bones or by refracturing and resetting them.

An enclosed rhinoplasty, where the incisions are all hidden within the nose, is the most commonly used technique.

All of these procedures, including correction of a deviated septum, may be performed under local anesthesia with IV sedation.

Surgical Procedure: Open Rhinoplasty
This technique is usually reserved for someone with very thin skin or someone who has undergone several rhinoplasties and has much scar tissue. In both cases, the surgeon has to see the problem bones and tissues directly to be able to correct the deformity.

Open rhinoplasty involves an incision on the lower part of the nose that extends into the nose. The skin of the nose is lifted up so that the surgeon can see the area. With meticulous cutting, the surgeon can change the shape of the cartilage and bone.

♦ Grafts using cartilage from the ear, nose or rib are sometimes used to enhance the tip or bridge of the nose.

♦ For nasal reconstruction, bone from a rib or the hip may be used to reconstruct severe deformities.

♦ Implants of solid silicone have been used to build up the dorsum (bridge of the nose) and tip. This is a popular procedure in Asia, but not in the United States.

After the Operation Because appearance depends on the precise nature of the operation, the results in one person may look completely different from those in another.

♦ When rhinoplasty involves cutting of the bone (osteotomy), there may be significant swelling afterwards. Black eyes are not uncommon.

♦ When only cartilage or tip work is involved, there is little postoperative swelling and you will look reasonably well.

♦ Most people wear a splint on the nose for about a week, which helps minimize swelling and helps the nasal bones heal.

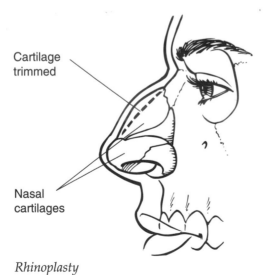

Cartilage trimmed

Nasal cartilages

Rhinoplasty

◆ It is not uncommon to have packing in the nose. Whether you have packing depends on the surgeon's technique and the amount of bleeding seen during the operation. The packing is not usually too uncomfortable, but you will have to breathe through your mouth until it is removed, usually within 24 to 48 hours.

CONTOURING THE CHIN AND CHEEKS

Plastic surgeons reshape many parts of the body with implanted materials, adding definition or highlighting particular areas. Sometimes, substances from your own body—bone and cartilage—are implanted. For reshaping areas of the face such as the cheek and chin, silicone solid implants are the most commonly used. Implants also enhance the angle of the jaw line and change the contour of the forehead.

Surgical Procedure Both chin and cheek implants are performed under local anesthesia with sedation.

For chin implants, the incision is made under the chin or inside the lower lip. After the tissues are lifted off the bone, the proper-sized implant is inserted and stitched into place. The incision is then sutured closed.

Cheek implants are placed through small incisions inside the upper lip, although they may be inserted through an external incision if you are also having a facelift or brow lift. Again, the tissues are lifted off the bone to create a space for the implant.

After the Operation With both procedures, you will have some swelling and numbness for the first week and possibly longer.
◆ Your diet will usually be restricted to soft foods and liquids for several days.
◆ You will be asked to rinse your mouth several times a day, perhaps with an antibiotic mouthwash, to prevent infection of the incisions inside your mouth.
◆ The stitches will usually dissolve within seven to 10 days.
◆ You may be able to return to work after a week. Discuss with the plastic surgeon any restrictions on your activities.
◆ A capsule of scar tissue may develop around the implant (capsular contracture). With either chin or cheek implants, however, even a very hard capsule should not cause any noticeable problem.

FLATTENING THE EARS

Protruding ears are common. What usually brings a patient to the cosmetic surgeon's office is the extent of the deviation. The operation designed to correct this condition is called an otoplasty.

Surgical Procedure Otoplasty recontours the cartilage of the ear, enabling it to bend backwards. This is usually done through a small incision behind the ear. The conchal cartilage is recontoured

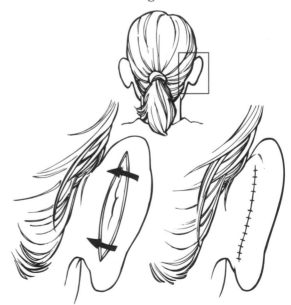

Flattening the ears

and sutured such that the ear is placed in a more aesthetic position. The ears are essentially pinned closer to the head. The results are immediate.

After the Operation You will be instructed to wear a headband—much like a sports sweatband—every night while asleep for about a month.
♦ Because the incision is behind the ear, it is well hidden. Most people have no visible scar.

LIPOSUCTION

Also called fat suction or suction lipectomy, liposuction has quickly become the most commonly performed cosmetic surgery in the United States.

Surgical Procedure Small incisions are made in the skin with a scalpel. A metal tube, or cannula, is inserted through the incisions into the distinct planes of tissue beneath the skin. This cannula is connected to an apparatus that essentially vacuums fat away.

By sweeping the cannula in these planes and removing the fat, the surgeon can recontour the face and the body. By varying the size of the cannula, the surgeon can recontour such delicate areas as the cheek, neck, knee and ankle as well as larger and broader areas such as the abdomen, hip, thigh and buttock.

Depending on the location of the fat and the amount to be removed, you may opt for local, regional or general anesthetic.
♦ In the operating room, you will be placed in a compressive garment. This will minimize swelling once the procedure is done.

Outpatient liposuction is limited by the amount of fat removed. Blood is also vacuumed up during liposuction. Studies have shown that 1,500 to 2,000 cc of fatty aspirate is the upper limit before a blood transfusion is considered.

The Need for Blood In a healthy person, removing 1,500 to 2,000 cc of fat may reduce the volume of blood enough to cause weakness, dizziness, lethargy and possible hypotension, or decrease in blood pressure. Orthostatic hypotension is a phenomenon where your blood pressure decreases when you stand up.
♦ IV fluids are always used during and after the procedure to maintain a healthy fluid level.
♦ If 1,500 to 2,000 cc of fatty aspirate are to be removed, you should be hospitalized overnight or have an autologous blood transfusion prepared. Plastic surgeons routinely set up an autologous blood supply when the anticipated fatty aspirate exceeds this limit.

Autologous blood is your own blood, given to a blood bank several weeks before the scheduled operation. This blood is kept on hand in case you need it during the operation or afterwards.

After the Operation You will be discharged only when you are able to walk around, your blood pressure is com-

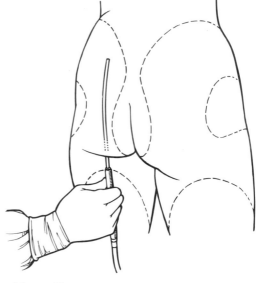

Liposuction

pletely stable and you have no symptoms of weakness, lethargy or dizziness.

◆ If there is any indication of orthostatic hypotension, you will be given more IV fluids and be observed for a longer time. Pain medications and general immobility can worsen orthostatic hypotension.

BREAST UPLIFT

Ptosis of the breasts is common with aging, particularly after giving birth and especially after multiple childbirths. The breasts lose some of their volume and tissues tend to atrophy, producing excess skin. The breasts then tend to droop.

A procedure called a mastopexy cor-

rects this problem, although the results may not be long-lasting and the procedure may leave noticeable scars. To provide additional volume, a saline breast implant is sometimes used in conjunction with the operation.

The incisions, possible scars and the need for an implant should all be discussed thoroughly with your cosmetic surgeon before the operation.

Surgical Procedure A mastopexy with and without a breast implant may be done on an outpatient basis under general anesthesia or local anesthesia with sedation.

The mastopexy lifts the nipple and areolar complex back to a more youthful position. An incision is made around

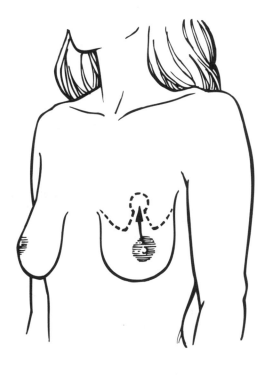
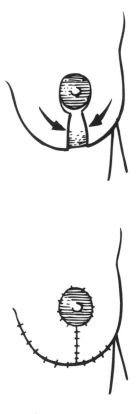

Breast uplift

the areola and down to the breast crease. Excess skin is removed, the nipple and areola are moved higher, and, with recontouring of the skin in relation to the breast volume, the shape of the breast is changed.

After the Operation You will need to wear a support bra for several weeks after the operation.
◆ Bruising and swelling are common over the first few days.
◆ It is wise to avoid sex for at least a week.
◆ You will have to avoid heavy lifting for several weeks.
◆ Discuss with your surgeon any other restrictions to your normal activities you should follow.

BREAST ENLARGEMENT

Breast implants have come under intense scrutiny because of problems with implants made of silicone gel. Because of potential problems with both silicone gel and polyurethane, these implants are no longer available for cosmetic purposes.

A saline implant, however, is still available for breast augmentation. A solid silicone shell contains saline, a saltwater solution commonly used in IV fluids. These implants have been used for many years to enhance the breast.

Again, thoroughly discuss all the pros and cons with your cosmetic surgeon before deciding to go ahead with the operation.

Part of this discussion should deal with where the implant will be placed. Today, the most common location is behind, rather than in front of, the main chest muscle (pectoralis major). This subpectoral approach appears to decrease the risk of developing a complication called symptomatic capsular contracture (*see* "After the Operation" below). It also appears to facilitate

mammographic screening of women with augmented breasts. With the soft breast tissue lying in front of not only the implant but the chest muscle itself, it is much easier to distinguish between breast tissue and the implant on a mammogram.

Surgical Procedure The implant is placed in various ways.
◆ The implant may be inserted through an incision either above or below the areola.
◆ The incision may be hidden in the crease where the breast meets the chest wall (inframammary crease).
◆ The incision may be made in the armpit (axillary incision), which also hides the scar.
◆ A newer technique is endoscopic placement of the breast implant through an incision either in the armpit or, more recently, in the navel. When performed by an experienced cosmetic surgeon, either route leaves a minimal scar.

After the Operation You will feel some soreness in the breast for several weeks after the operation. There may also be some burning sensation in the nipples.
◆ Stitches will be removed after about a week, at which time you may return to showering or bathing normally.
◆ Discuss with your surgeon when you may return to work and resume your normal activities.
◆ An infection may develop around the implant, although this is rare.
◆ It is also rare for the implant to leak or break. When a saline implant ruptures, the salt water is absorbed by the body. The shell has to be removed and a new implant inserted.
◆ The most common complication is developing a capsular contracture. The body's natural response is to surround the foreign substance it considers an invader. This inflammatory response causes a capsule around the implant,

which may harden and cause several symptoms, including an uncomfortable firmness. A capsular contracture occurs in almost everyone, but does not cause any symptoms in most women. If the capsule is extremely hard and symptomatic, the capsule should be removed (capsulectomy) and the implant changed or moved to a new position.

SCAR REVISIONS

Sometimes the body is very aggressive in healing a wound and an unsightly scar is the result. Such a scar is oriented in such a way that the scar tissue is heaped up in an irregular contour. Depending on where such scars are located, they may be very undesirable. They can be revised, however, by a variety of techniques, including non-surgical methods.

Most scars tend to improve with time, so scar revision should not be performed until after the scar is completely matured and has improved as much as naturally possible. This often requires up to a year of observation, although a scar revision may be done earlier if the scar is in a particularly sensitive area, such as near the eye.

A scar revision cannot guarantee an improvement. Some people have intrinsic wound-healing properties that produce hypertrophic scars or keloids. Hypertrophic scars are thick and red, although they usually flatten out over time. Keloids are thick, dark and irregular bits of scar tissue that may grow beyond the incision.

Each scar must be carefully assessed. Some parts of the body heal differently with revisions, and some parts are particularly prone to keloid formation.

Non-Surgical Techniques Several non-surgical techniques are used to combat a scar.
◆ Steroids are injected into the scar, to produce some shrinkage.
◆ A pressure garment is worn or a silicone wafer is applied.
◆ Dermabrasion (rubbing away the top layers of the skin with an instrument much like a wire brush), tattooing, laser treatment and chemical peels may be applied to a superficial scar.

Surgical Procedure The scar tissue may simply be cut out. The wound is closed with a meticulous plastics closure under no tension.

A Z-plasty is often performed. This involves removing the old scar, then making two new incisions on either side. This creates small skin flaps that are rotated to cover the original incision site. In this way, the surgeon reorients the direction of the scar to minimize tension on the wound.

HAIR TRANSPLANTS

Hair transplants are much in the news and advertising these days. Hair transplantation involves anything from plugs, microplugs and grafts to the microsurgical transfer of other areas of the scalp over to the bald regions.

The various techniques must be individualized, so you should consult physicians well experienced in this field.

When you see a plastic surgeon, he or she will explain all the options and ask about any family history of baldness, about your own experience and what you expect from a hair replacement procedure.

Surgical Procedures Plugs are small, round grafts of hair-bearing tissue that are "punched" out of the back of the scalp and replanted into punched-out holes in the bald areas. The donor sites are usually stitched closed, and a bandage holds the grafts in place. The procedure is usually done under local anesthesia.

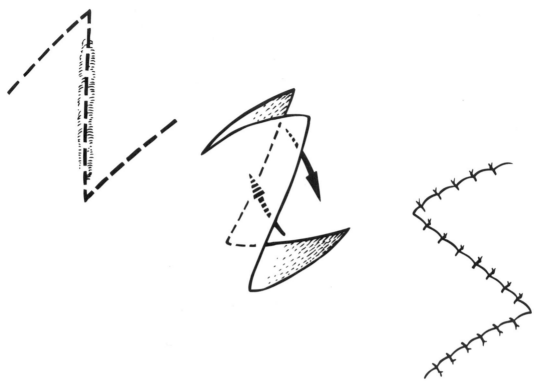

Z-plasty

Filling in a large area of baldness may require several sessions over many months. Even smaller plugs (miniplugs and microplugs) are used to fill in the spaces between the larger grafts or to give your hair a more natural look. Plugs are positioned to maintain your natural angle of hair growth.

◆ With scalp reduction, a patch of bald skin is cut out of the crown. The remaining skin is loosened, then the sides are brought together and stitched closed.

◆ With tissue expansion, a balloon-type device is placed under the scalp on the sides of the head. Over time, the device is gradually inflated to stretch the skin. Bald areas are then covered with the expanded tissue.

◆ Hair weaving and similar techniques make the hair-bearing region appear fuller and denser.

◆ The most aggressive type of hair transplantation is microsurgical free tissue transfer. This is appropriate for only a small minority of patients. A region of hair-bearing scalp is removed with its blood vessels. It is then transplanted to the bald regions of the scalp and the blood vessels are reconnected with the aid of a microscope.

After the Operation There may be some pain after plugs are inserted, although many people do not find the procedure uncomfortable. The bandage will usually be removed two days after the operation. Any stitches will be removed in a week.

◆ It will take three months for normal

circulation to return to the scalp after the plugs are transplanted.

◆ After tissue expansion and scalp reduction, you may feel a little tightness in the scalp. This usually fades quickly, but if the skin is very tight the scar may widen. Bandages are removed after the first week and the stitches taken out in about 10 days. The scar is barely visible after the first two weeks.

◆ After any hair replacement procedure, it will take several weeks to gradually return to your normal activities. Any vigorous activity may damage grafts and stitches or increase the blood flow to the head, causing bleeding.

QUESTIONS TO ASK YOUR PLASTIC AND RECONSTRUCTIVE SURGEON

◆ Are you Board-certified in plastic surgery?

◆ How many of these procedures have you done?

◆ How noticeable will my scars be?

◆ Are there surgical alternatives to the procedure you recommend?

◆ How long will healing take and what complications should I look for?

◆ How long does it take to get the best results? And how long will they last?

15
ORTHOPEDIC SURGERY

David W. Lowenberg, MD

Orthopedics is the field of medicine concerned with correcting or curing diseases of the bones, joints and other parts of the skeletal system.

Orthopedic surgery lends itself particularly well to outpatient surgical procedures because it focuses on the limbs and the abdominal cavity isn't involved in any way, so patients may begin eating and drinking again the same day as the surgery. And because only one limb is usually involved, patients can still move around and carry on with normal activities, although a sling, splint or shoulder immobilizer may be necessary after arm surgery and some immobilization of the leg and/or crutches may be necessary after surgery to the knee, foot or ankle.

TYPES OF ORTHOPEDIC PROCEDURES

Most orthopedic procedures fall into three general categories.

Percutaneous The first category involves procedures that are performed completely via small incisions through the skin (percutaneously). These procedures are considered minimally invasive.

The most common example is arthroscopy, which means to view the joint. Arthroscopic surgery is now the most frequently performed orthopedic operation in the United States. It is performed with the aid of an arthroscope, a thin stainless steel–encased tube with fiberoptic elements inside. The arthroscope serves as a lens. Attached to the arthroscope is a light source, to illuminate the body cavity being inspected, and a small video camera.

The surgeon makes a small incision, places the arthroscope through the incision into the body, usually inside a joint, then manipulates it as necessary while viewing what he or she is doing on a video monitor. With the arthroscope, procedures that previously required several days of hospitalization may now be performed as outpatient surgery.

There are many benefits of arthroscopy.

◆ The arthroscope enables access to areas of a joint that are otherwise difficult to reach.

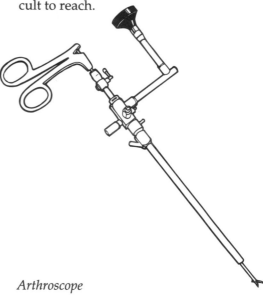

Arthroscope

◆ Since an optical system is used, the area being treated is magnified and small objects are seen much more clearly than with the unaided eye.

◆ Since the incisions are very small, there is less pain and scarring, which usually leads to easier rehabilitation.

◆ The 1/4 in. (5 mm) incisions normal for arthroscopy leave a much better cosmetic result.

Open Procedures These are what most people usually think of as "an operation." A long incision is made in the skin and the area and the procedure are seen directly by the surgeon. Procedures not involving joints are commonly done this way.

Combination The last category involves operations performed with both percutaneous and open techniques. These procedures rely on technological advances such as fluoroscopy and arthroscopy to allow surgery in a less invasive fashion and with smaller incisions than was previously possible.

A now common example is arthroscopically assisted reconstruction of the anterior cruciate ligament in the knee, a ligament that athletes commonly injure. All the work inside the knee is done percutaneously with the arthroscope and only small incisions are needed to attach the reconstructed ligament to the bone.

Certain biopsy procedures are done with the aid of fluoroscopy and special biopsy instruments.

PLANNING FOR YOUR SURGERY

It cannot be overemphasized that you fully discuss with your surgeon not only what will be involved in your operation but also what will happen afterwards. You will then be better able to plan and prepare, all of which

will lessen the stress of the surgical experience.

◆ Ask your surgeon how long you will have to use crutches or other aids.

◆ It is helpful to obtain the crutches before surgery so you can learn how to use them in advance.

The Need for Rehabilitation One feature that differentiates outpatient orthopedic procedures from other forms of surgery is the need for rehabilitation. This usually involves a program of muscle strengthening or joint range of motion exercises, which often requires supervision by a physiotherapist.

It is usually beneficial to see the physiotherapist before the operation, so the therapist can teach you the exercises involved in the rehabilitation program when it is easier for the limb involved to do the exercises properly. The therapist can also maximize muscle strength and conditioning so that the deconditioning that often occurs when a limb is immobilized postoperatively will be minimized.

REMOVING PLATES AND SCREWS

Broken bones are often repaired with stainless steel plates, which have holes in them to accommodate screws that fix the plate to the bone. This is common for fractures of the ankle and of the two bones of the forearm, the radius and ulna.

After the fracture has healed, your surgeon may decide that the hardware should be taken out. This is often an outpatient procedure.

Surgical Procedure The operation is usually performed with general or regional anesthesia. The incision made to insert the plate is reopened and the hardware removed. This can be trickier than it sounds, because the surgeon may have to cut through tougher scar tissue, which can be quite difficult.

After the Operation The extremity involved often has to be immobilized for a while to allow the screw holes to fill in with new bone. This is necessary because the screw holes may be a site of refracture.

◆ The surgeon will provide you with an appropriate plan for protecting and rehabilitating your limb. In the case of the leg and ankle, this usually means that you will have to use crutches.

SHOULDER ARTHROSCOPY

Until the last decade, outpatient procedures around the shoulder were limited to simple biopsy or excising the outer end of the clavicle for arthritis of the acromioclavicular joint. This procedure is still commonly performed for symptomatic arthritis of the acromioclavicular joint. But, mainly because of arthroscopy, many more shoulder procedures are now performed as outpatient surgery.

Before the Operation When surgery is recommended for a shoulder ailment, there are several questions you should ask your surgeon.

◆ It is first important to know whether your shoulder will have to be immobilized after the operation. This information will allow you to better plan your rehabilitation. You might require assistance at home with preparing meals, bathing and housecleaning. This is especially true if surgery is planned for your dominant arm (for instance, your right if you are right-handed).

◆ If your shoulder does have to be immobilized, ask whether the immobilizer may be removed for short periods for activities such as bathing. (Also be aware that when an arm is placed in an immobilizer, it is not uncommon for the hand and wrist to become swollen because of the prolonged dependent position of the hand and forearm.)

◆ Physical therapy is often a necessary part of rehabilitation after shoulder surgery, so ask your surgeon the details of the rehabilitation program, as well as when physical therapy should be started.

◆ Some shoulder procedures may result in a loss of shoulder motion, so ask whether a significant loss in motion might be expected and whether this will be permanent or temporary.

Surgical Procedure: Arthroscopy Arthroscopy of the shoulder is performed under either general or regional anesthesia. You will be positioned either in a semi-sitting position (as if you were lying in a beach chair) or on your side with the affected side up.

The shoulder joint may be seen completely through two or three incisions, each measuring about 1/3 in. (8 mm). Using the arthroscope for visualization and guidance, the surgeon will insert small hand instruments and motorized shaving instruments into the joint space.

Common procedures involve cutting or trimming (debriding) a part of the joint or the interior of the joint capsule. These procedures often successfully relieve certain painful conditions.

Surgical Procedure: Arthroscopy for Rotator Cuff Tendonitis The most common arthroscopic procedure of the shoulder treats rotator cuff tendonitis.

The rotator cuff consists of the tendons of four muscles: the subscapularis, supraspinatus, infraspinatus and teres minor. These form a hood over the head of the humerus at the top of the joint. The function of the rotator cuff is to hold the head of the humerus against the glenoid, which is the flat, fixed part

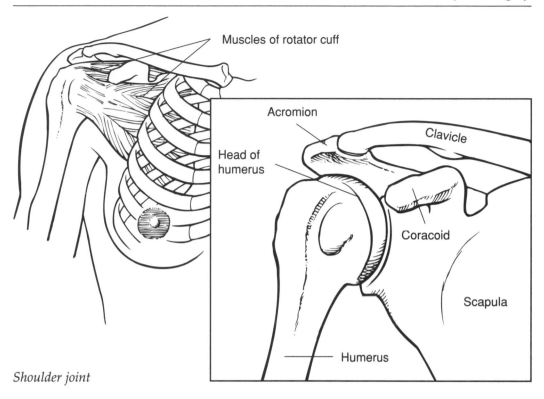

Muscles of rotator cuff

Acromion

Clavicle

Head of
humerus

Coracoid

Scapula

Humerus

Shoulder joint

of the shoulder joint. By holding the head of the humerus against the glenoid, the rotator cuff allows the larger deltoid muscle to raise the arm.

People who have completely torn their rotator cuffs have great difficulty raising their arm because the humeral head is no longer stabilized against the glenoid. With no fixed point of rotation, the deltoid tends to lift the humerus upward without letting the head roll against the glenoid as it should.

Rotator cuff tendonitis is also referred to as bursitis of the shoulder. This involves irritation to the rotator cuff usually because of the abutment of the cuff against the lip of the acromion, where the collar bone attaches to the shoulder.

The surgeon places the arthroscope in the bursal sac between the rotator cuff and the acromion, and then uses motorized instruments and burrs to cut the anterior lip of the acromion. This

eliminates the impingement on the rotator cuff.

After the Operation Upon discharge, you will be given pain medications.

♦ Your arm will often be in a sling or shoulder immobilizer.

♦ The rehabilitation program recommended by your surgeon will usually involve progressive activities to restore arm and shoulder motion.

Surgical Procedure: Dislocated Shoulder People suffering from recurring dislocations of the shoulder have usually been treated with an open operation. But this common shoulder ailment is now occasionally being treated surgically on an outpatient basis.

The procedure uses the arthroscope to assist in surgically stabilizing the dislocated shoulder. Stitches are placed under arthroscopic control.

This is not always feasible. Only your surgeon can decide whether you are a candidate for this procedure rather than the more conventional open surgical treatment.

THE ELBOW AND FOREARM

The elbow is an unusual joint because it allows for two types of motion.
◆ The articulation between the olecranon and the medial condyle of the humerus allows for flexion and extension of the elbow. This is the motion people most commonly associate with elbow function.
◆ The articulation between the head of the radius and the lateral condyle of the humerus allows for rotation of the forearm and hand. This rotation is essential for functional use of the hand.

A limited number of outpatient operations are performed on the elbow. As with other joints, arthroscopy may be done either to remove loose bodies or to treat an array of rarer conditions.

Before the Operation Ask your surgeon
◆ How long must the elbow be immobilized?
◆ What arm activities are permitted during the recovery period so I may plan for any assistance needed at home?

Find out about any lifting restrictions during the rehabilitation period and have your surgeon explain the time frame for regaining elbow motion. This will help you gauge your progress during rehabilitation.

Surgical Procedure: Tennis Elbow About 90 percent of tennis elbow cases—called lateral epicondylitis—are managed with splinting, job modification, the use of non-steroidal anti-inflammatory drugs and the judicious use of cortisone injections. Someone whose elbow doesn't respond to these therapies may be treated with outpatient surgery.

Through a small incision, the three extensor tendons originating at the lateral epicondyle of the humerus are released. The extensor muscles still

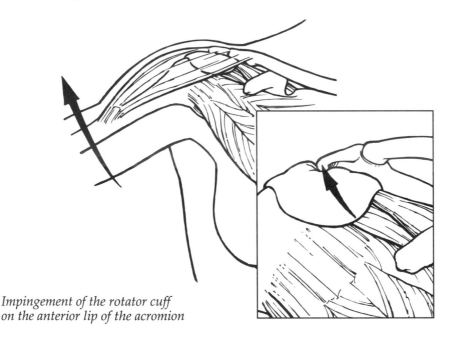

Impingement of the rotator cuff on the anterior lip of the acromion

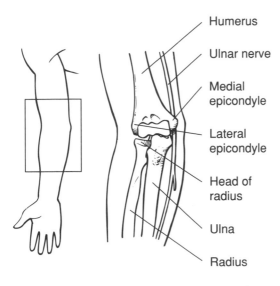

Humerus

Ulnar nerve

Medial
epicondyle

Lateral
epicondyle

Head of
radius

Ulna

Radius

Elbow joint

function normally, so this procedure does not cause any problems with wrist or hand function.

After the Operation Prolonged immobilization is rarely necessary.
♦ Rehabilitation after this procedure is usually several weeks.

Surgical Procedure: Cubital Tunnel Syndrome Another common procedure performed around the elbow is transposition of the ulnar nerve. This is done for a condition called cubital tunnel syndrome, which involves compression and entrapment of the ulnar nerve as it passes behind the medial epicondyle of the humerus.

The ulnar nerve provides sensation to the little finger and one half of the ring finger. It also supplies nerves to most of the small muscles in the hand. People with cubital tunnel syndrome usually complain of tingling and numbness around their little finger. They also occasionally notice weakness in spreading their fingers and some weakness in

grasp with the little and ring fingers.

Before surgery, your surgeon may obtain nerve conduction studies of the ulnar nerve. This test measures the speed of an electrical impulse traveling along the nerve and will help confirm that the ulnar nerve is being compressed.

The procedure involves making an incision on the inner side of the elbow. The surgeon moves the ulnar nerve, which sits behind the elbow, to in front of the elbow. This takes the tension off the ulnar nerve and reduces or eliminates symptoms.

After the Operation
♦ Ask your surgeon how long the elbow must be immobilized, and what activities of the arm are permitted during the recovery period. You can then better plan for any assistance needed at home.
♦ Find out about any lifting restrictions during the rehabilitation period.
♦ Find out from your surgeon the time frame for regaining elbow motion. This will help you to gauge your progress during the rehabilitation period.

KNEE ARTHROSCOPY

Knee arthroscopy used to be limited to simple visualization of the knee joint to help orthopedic surgeons make a diagnosis. Technological improvements have made it possible to perform surgical procedures with the use of the arthroscope.

The knee is well suited for arthroscopy because there is very little soft tissue between the joint and the skin. The arthroscope also allows access to areas in the joint that are normally difficult to see even when large incisions are made.

For most procedures, three incisions, each measuring 1/3 in. (8 mm), are made near the knee. Some procedures require one or two additional incisions.

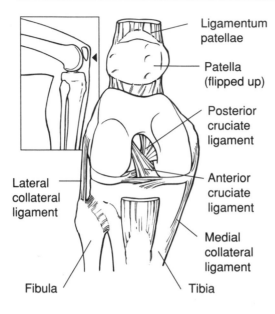

Knee joint

Surgical Procedure: Removing a Torn Meniscus The most common procedure is removal of part or all of the medial or lateral meniscus. The menisci are C-shaped pieces of cartilage on the inner (medial) and outer (lateral) parts of the knee that function as shock absorbers between the femur and tibia. These structures may tear either because of an injury or because of simple wear.

A torn meniscus causes pain on that side of the knee and may also cause clicking and popping with knee motion. Occasionally, a large tear in the meniscus causes the knee to lock in a flexed position. This sometimes requires an urgent visit to the orthopedist to unlock the joint manually. A torn meniscus may also cause repeated episodes of knee swelling.

Using the arthroscope for visualization and a host of small instruments, the surgeon can remove the torn piece of meniscus with great precision. If the torn meniscus has broken free within the joint, it, along with any other loose bodies, is easily removed.

After the Operation Rehabilitation is quite rapid after this procedure.
◆ Often your surgeon will allow you to begin bearing weight on the operated limb soon after surgery.
◆ Immobilization of the knee is generally not necessary, and range of motion exercises can be started immediately.
◆ About one week after surgery, you may begin a muscle-strengthening program to help speed recovery.
◆ Your orthopedic surgeon will direct your rehabilitation and postoperative care.

Surgical Procedure: Repairing a Torn Meniscus In younger patients, it is sometimes possible to repair the torn meniscus with the aid of the arthroscope. An additional incision measuring about 1 in. (2.5 cm) is often required to allow the safe placement of stitches as well as tying of the stitches snugly against the joint capsule.

This is a technically demanding procedure. There are various ways of doing it, and your surgeon will pick the best method of repair for the type of tear involved. The procedure is best suited for simple tears on the outside edge of the meniscus, because only the outside one-third has a blood supply. The central two-thirds of the meniscus receives all its nutrition from the joint fluid. As might be expected, tissue with a blood supply heals better than tissue without.

After the Operation The postoperative course for a meniscal repair is different than that for removal of the meniscus.
◆ A much longer recovery and rehabilitation are required.
◆ Most orthopedic surgeons require that you use crutches and put no weight on the affected leg for six weeks.
◆ Many surgeons also immobilize the leg in a cast or brace.

Surgical Procedure: Arthritis of the Knee Many patients suffering from early arthritis of the knee have benefited from an arthroscopy of the knee to clean out the joint. Damaged parts may be smoothed out or removed, which may reduce some of the pain as well as the mechanical catching and clicking of the joint associated with arthritis.

Although the procedure may provide relief from symptoms for one to three years, it does not reverse or alter the progress of arthritis.

Surgical Procedure: Reconstructing the Anterior Cruciate Ligament The anterior cruciate ligament is a large structure in the center of the knee that provides joint stability by preventing the femur from sliding against the tibia.

A torn anterior cruciate ligament may be reconstructed through very small incisions, using the arthroscope for visualization. The procedure restores functional stability to the knee.

When this ligament tears, the ends are frayed and cannot be fixed, so other tissue has to be used. Some surgeons use tissue from around the knee, while others prefer the use of allograft tissue. Allograft means that the tissue is taken from a healthy person who has died, usually in an accident. This tissue is screened and processed to make it safe for reimplantation, and there is no threat of infection from the donor. Using allograft tissue means that you don't have to sacrifice any of your own tendons or ligaments to make the new anterior cruciate ligament.

Ask your surgeon what tissue she or he is using for your reconstruction and discuss the pros and cons.

After the Operation Rehabilitation takes several months and usually requires a great deal of compliance and work on your part.
◆ A period of bracing is usually required.
◆ Depending on the type of reconstruction, your orthopedic surgeon might also require that you use crutches to avoid putting weight on the affected leg.
◆ At some point during rehabilitation, you will start a vigorous exercise program, both to regain full knee range of motion and to restore strength to the quadriceps and hamstring muscles.
◆ Care must be taken to protect the reconstruction for one year, which is how long it takes for new blood vessels to fully grow into the new ligament.

ANKLE ARTHROSCOPY

With the advent of improved optics and smaller-diameter arthroscopes and instruments, arthroscopy of the ankle may now be performed to remove loose bodies, stabilize chronic ligament injuries and clean out an arthritic joint. This is usually done through two or three 1/4 in. (5 mm) incisions. Rehabilitation is quite rapid.

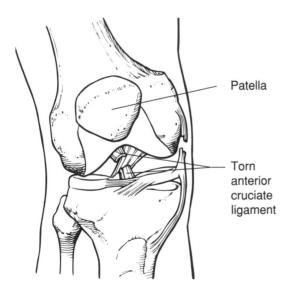

Patella

Torn anterior cruciate ligament

Torn anterior cruciate ligament

BUNIONS

Bunions are bony growths on the outside of the base of the big toe. There are two types.

◆ The most common type develops during adult life, usually as a result of shoe wear. They occur much more frequently in women than in men because of women's use of narrow-tipped shoes with high heels.

◆ The other, and much rarer, type develops during adolescence and is usually an inherited condition.

Many people have bunion deformities that are painless, and most people with painful bunions are successfully treated simply by wearing shoes with a wide toe box.

A bunion correction should not be performed for cosmetic reasons. The only reason for treatment is relief of pain that cannot be controlled by modifying footwear. If you have a painful bunion and your pain is not managed by wearing wider shoes, consult with your orthopedic surgeon about whether you would benefit from corrective surgery.

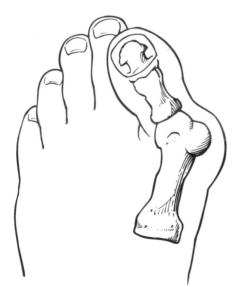

Bunion

Surgical Procedure There are many surgical procedures for treating bunion deformities, all of them involving the removal of the bony prominence. The second part of the procedure involves correcting the twisted and angulated big toe. Sometimes this is accomplished by tightening and rebalancing the soft tissue around the big toe. In other cases, the bones around the toe have to be broken and reset to achieve a proper correction.

Your orthopedic surgeon will decide on which procedure will work best for you based on your age, degree of deformity and x-ray findings.

After the Operation It is important to follow your surgeon's instructions carefully.

◆ A good result partially depends on correct immobilization, splinting or wrapping of the toe to prevent a recurrence. Usually such care has to be continued for six weeks to allow the bone and soft tissues to heal in the right position.

◆ Most orthopedic surgeons require their patients to wear a special firm-soled shoe, open at the toes, for six weeks after surgery.

◆ To help prevent infection and wound-healing problems, follow your surgeon's instructions about elevating your foot until the wound is completely healed and the stitches are removed.

◆ Do not return to your old shoe-wear habits. The bunion deformity may recur if you go back to wearing narrow, pointed shoes.

HAMMER TOES

Hammer toes are deformities of the four small toes. Over time, the toes begin to claw. This condition may develop after some injury to the leg or foot, because of improper shoe wear or as a secondary effect of a bunion deformity.

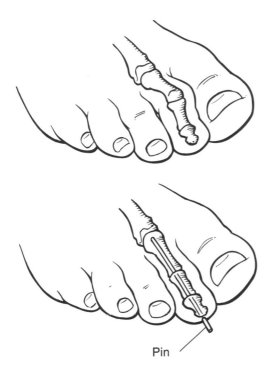

Pin

Hammer toe procedure

Painful calluses often develop on the tips of the toes because of the awkward position of the toe while walking. Calluses also develop on the tops of the toes because of the constant rubbing and irritation of the toes against the shoe.

Surgical Procedure Hammer toes are treated successfully by releasing the tight structures around the toe, then pinning the toe in an acceptable posi-

tion with a thin stainless steel pin. The tendon on the bottom of the foot that causes the toe to flex occasionally must be cut.

After the correction, you won't be able to wiggle the affected toe with any force, but this will not alter the way you walk. The benefit of the correction far outweighs any problems because you will once again be able to walk and wear shoes without pain.

After the Operation The stainless steel fixation pin is usually left in the toe for six weeks, then removed during a follow-up office visit with your orthopedic surgeon.

♦ A special shoe, like that worn after bunion surgery, must be used for six weeks after surgery.

♦ The fixation pin is often left sticking out of the skin at the tip of the toe, so you will have to take special care to avoid hitting the pin and to keep the pin clean to prevent infection.

QUESTIONS TO ASK YOUR ORTHOPEDIC SURGEON

♦ How soon after my surgery may I bathe or shower and get my wound wet?
♦ How long after surgery on my leg may I begin walking?
♦ Will I need to take antibiotics after surgery?
♦ When may I return to work?

16
HAND SURGERY

Robert E. Markison, MD, FACS

The human hand is a part of the body involved in vocation, avocation, communication and affection. People are naturally concerned about even small problems in their hands because of the importance of the hand in work and play.

The domain of hand surgery encompasses both non-surgical and surgical remedies for problems that may be present at birth, are gradually acquired

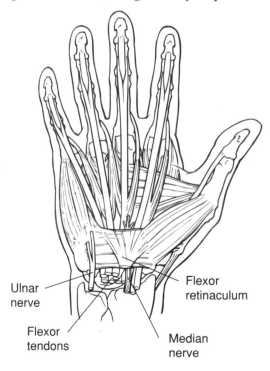

Ulnar nerve

Flexor tendons

Flexor retinaculum

Median nerve

Anatomy of the hand

or are caused by acute injuries and infections.

SPECIAL TECHNIQUES OF HAND SURGERY

One of the pioneers of hand surgery, Sterling Bunnell, referred to the hand as the "Swiss watch of the body." He also emphasized the importance of a bloodless surgical field, saying that a surgeon cannot "operate in an inkwell." By this he meant that even minimal staining of tissues with blood during a hand operation may obscure critically important and closely packed anatomy.

The major tenets of hand surgery are gentle handling of the patient and gentle handling of tissues without any blood loss.

You and Your Surgeon The hand is a demanding body part to work on. Your surgeon should have substantial experience and should also plan to stand by you during the entire course of healing. Hands often heal slowly, especially in cool-handed people. Some operations require a year or more to achieve the most benefit.

Whenever an operation might be necessary, discuss with your surgeon all the non-surgical and surgical options. Rapport with your surgeon is very important, especially because follow-up may span anywhere from six months to two years. The surgeon will make a diagnosis and devise a treatment plan based on an understanding of mutual goals.

Achieving fine results in hand surgery is truly a team effort, involving a great deal of cooperation between patient and surgeon.

Standard Practices Many procedures are done in an office under local anesthesia. The surgeon will wear magnifying eyeglasses, called loupes, to see all the structures involved.

For a minor hand procedure not requiring an anesthesiologist, you can expect the following sequence.

◆ For treatment of even the most minor hand problems, it is best that you lie face up in a comfortable position with the hand away from your body on a padded table or stand. Fainting may occur if you are sitting upright.

◆ If a minor procedure is to be performed, a tourniquet is applied either to the arm above the elbow or to the near side of the forearm below the elbow. A digit tourniquet may be used if the problem is at the thumb or fingertips.

◆ The arm or forearm tourniquet will not be inflated until the limb has been elevated, the skin has been painted with an antiseptic solution and the local anesthesia, or regional nerve block with local anesthesia, has been given.

◆ Sterile draping will be applied to your forearm or hand. A vertical drape is placed so that you will not be able to observe the procedure.

◆ The surgeon will inflate the arm or forearm tourniquet or apply the digit tourniquet. The surgeon will keep close track of time so that there is no undue discomfort. Under local anesthesia, a tourniquet may safely be left in place about 20 or 30 minutes.

◆ The operation is done very gently and the skin wound is generally closed with an easily removable suture or one that your body will absorb. With children, most operations are done with

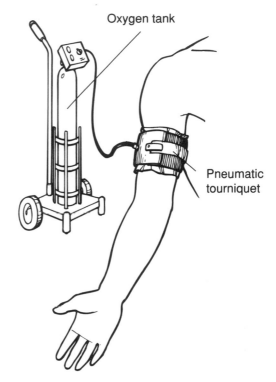

Oxygen tank

Pneumatic tourniquet

Tourniquet

absorbable sutures to avoid the discomfort of taking out the stitches later on.

◆ The tourniquet is deflated and a dressing is applied, which will often include a layer of plaster for support and protection. Sometimes the tourniquet is deflated before the wound is closed. This will depend on the nature and location of the procedure and the surgeon's preference.'

◆ You will be given instructions about keeping the limb elevated above the level of the heart (left midchest), elevating it on a pillow when you are lying down or keeping it up on a stack of pillows when you're sitting up. It is important to keep the hand above the level of the heart for two to four days after surgery to avoid swelling or throbbing discomfort.

◆ You will be given telephone numbers so you can reach the surgeon should you have any questions or problems.

◆ You will be given pain medicine for use as needed. In some cases a day or two of antibiotics will be appropriate.

◆ Follow-up will sometimes be within two or three days, but more often within five or seven days for a dressing change and possible application of a cast, a splint or a light, simple dressing. Sutures will be removed in 10 to 14 days.

◆ In most cases, you will be responsible for remobilizing your hand. In some cases, hand therapy by a physical or occupational therapist will be necessary for four to six weeks.

GETTING THE BEST RESULTS

If you are going to obtain the best possible result from hand surgery, there are certain guidelines to bear in mind.

◆ General medical conditions should be under control before surgery, including blood glucose control in diabetics, thyroid control in patients with hyper- or hypothyroidism, blood pressure control for hypertensives and so on.

◆ Don't smoke. Nicotine is a powerful constrictor of small blood vessels and will shut off the circulation to structures that are healing and most need the blood supply for nutrients.

◆ Refrain from drinking alcohol, which impairs the early phases of wound healing.

◆ If you have cool hands, wear fingerless cotton or wool gloves.

◆ Plan ahead for surgery. If you live alone and will not be able to cook for a week or two, stock up on frozen meals.

◆ Relax, and understand that healing in the hand takes a great deal of time. Stress and scarring seem to go together. Unduly tense patients tend to get more scarring, which leads to less than ideal results.

◆ Patients who eat well do well. Eating well means consuming a good deal of fresh produce.

◆ Anyone who is markedly obese and has time before surgery should take on an appropriate weight loss program so the limb will bear less of a load. Obese patients do not do particularly well with any type of hand surgery because of the loading of the hand and wrist by extra fat on the limb plus the demands placed on the hand by a good deal of weight from the shoulder to the fingertips.

ANESTHESIA

Local anesthesia is sufficient for simple exploration of traumatic wounds, the removal of superficial skin lesions, repair of tendons in some regions on the top side of the hand and drainage of minor infections of the fingertips or skin.

Regional Anesthesia Many operations require intravenous regional anesthesia. A tourniquet will be applied to your arm or forearm, then an IV will be placed in the top surface of the hand or sometimes in the wrist or forearm. This IV will be used to inject local anesthesia.

The limb is then elevated and a rubber bandage called an esmarch is wrapped snugly from fingertips to tourniquet to push the blood from the limb back into the general circulation. The tourniquet is inflated, the esmarch removed and local anesthesia injected to fill the veins. This will provide an excellent anesthetic for operations that last up to about an hour. Sometimes an IV regional block will work for up to two hours.

An IV in the opposite hand will provide sedation. Some common anesthetic agents provide not only calm but also amnesia about the surgical experience. You will often not remember any details of the procedure.

In rare cases, the anesthetic causes minimal side effects, such as a slight dizziness or a metallic taste in the mouth.

General Anesthesia General anesthesia is used for operations lasting longer than one and a half to two hours. General anesthesia for upper limb operations need not be deep because the surgeon will frequently block the peripheral nerves with local anesthesia to ensure comfort.

In all cases, a long-acting local anesthesia is injected into the edges of the incision. This will provide pain relief for two to eight hours. Many patients will not need to take any pain medications after surgery, provided they elevate the limb.

TENDON INJURIES

Tendon injuries in the hand, often involving glass or knife wounds, are common. In the case of glass wounds, the glass is found on an x-ray of the hand 90 percent of the time. The glass is removed at the time of tendon repair.

If the tendon injury involves the top of the knuckle joints or the midportion of the top of the hand, the injury is sometimes repaired under local anesthesia in an emergency or operating room.

Local anesthesia is not advisable for tendon injuries on the palm side of the hand, at the wrist level or along the forearm. Tendon injuries at these levels are a challenge because muscle-tendon units act much like rubber bands. Once they are divided, the near side of the tendon tends to spring back into the hand, wrist or forearm, which requires a slightly more extensive procedure for retrieval of the tendon stump for repair.

The most challenging tendon repairs are in the palm or out into the fingers. This is because of the proximity of tendons to each other and to other vital structures such as nerves and arteries

and also because tendons run through tunnels, or sheaths, which begin at the far creases on the palm and end at the final joints of the fingers and thumb.

Surgical Procedure Repairs in these regions must be done by experienced hand surgeons. Any significant tendon repair in the hand, wrist or forearm should be done by a surgeon with substantial experience in upper limb tendon repair and who can follow the patient closely for about six months.

Tendons are generally repaired with non-absorbable inert sutures. Such repairs ensure proper tendon strength while allowing good gliding of a tendon relative to its neighboring structures.

After the Operation Your hand will be immobilized for three to four weeks after a tendon repair.
◆ As the hand is gradually remobilized, do not do any power gripping for at least two or three months. Tendon healing continues for six months to one year.
◆ Initially, the tendon will stick, or scar, to surrounding structures, but will gradually re-establish its path of glide.

Follow-up Remobilization may involve close follow-up two or three times a week, with passive motion of the digit by the surgeon and/or hand therapist.
◆ It may also involve a technique in which a rubber band is applied to the top surface of the fingernail using a hook that is glued onto the nail. The rubber band is fastened (particularly in cases of flexor tendon injury) to a safety pin over the wrist area of a plaster dressing. You will be instructed to straighten out the finger and then let the finger fall as the rubber band pulls the finger into a flexed position. This permits gliding of the tendon repair so that the repair site does not get stuck to surrounding structures.
◆ Early mobilization techniques must be

carefully supervised by the surgeon. There is a small risk of rupture of the repair with such techniques. Success depends on a great deal of care in applying the dressing and excellent cooperation between patient and surgeon.

♦ No surgeon can guarantee complete return of function after a tendon repair, because the tendency to scar varies substantially.

NERVE INJURIES

Nerves in the upper limb have two properties: they may be sensory nerves responsible for feeling and feedback of temperature, pain, position and so on, or they may be motor nerves responsible for directing the movement of muscle tendons.

♦ The radial nerve is a pure sensory nerve in the upper limb giving feeling to the top surface of the thumb and the index and middle fingers.

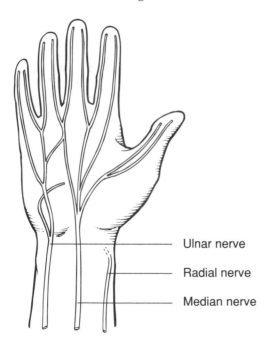

Nerves of the hand

♦ The ulnar nerve is a mixed sensory-motor nerve giving feeling to the ring and little fingers, and giving motion to some finger flexors in the forearm and to 15 of the 20 small muscles in the hand.

♦ The median nerve is called the eye of the hand because it gives feeling to the pads of the thumb, the index and middle fingers and part of the ring finger. This is a critically important nerve for feeding back the sense of touch.

Surgical Procedure Nerve repair is demanding. A microscope may have to be used for small nerves, for untidy nerve injuries and for nerve injuries with gaps requiring grafting of nerve segments from other parts of the body. Nerve graft donor sites include small nerves that cross the inside of the elbow, the sural nerve from the lower leg and ankle area, and sometimes other sites.

Stitches many times smaller than a human hair are used to sew the nerve bundles together.

After the Operation Nerves are some of the slowest-healing structures in the body, regenerating at a rate of about 1/32 in. (1 mm) per day, which amounts to about 1 in. (2.5 cm) per month. If a nerve is divided at mid-forearm and must regrow to the fingertips, it could take 16 months simply to migrate to the tip and it might be two to two and a half years before the final result can be evaluated. This can be a frustratingly slow process during which time you may lack feeling and muscle action.

♦ Nerve repairs are generally immobilized for about two weeks. Sometimes partial nerve injuries are mobilized earlier. Hand therapy is occasionally necessary.

♦ It is important to avoid burn injuries and crush injuries to the relatively insensate part of the hand on the far side of a nerve repair. It is also important to keep the hand flexible pending re-innervation of large or small muscle groups. A stiff hand will not work well at all even though the muscle may regain its action.

Follow-up For one or two years, the surgeon will gently test for a sign called Tinel's sign. He or she will tap on the far edge of the nerve's territory and then gently tap closer and closer, usually with a pencil eraser, to see if there is any tingling sensation. The Tinel's sign should advance from near to far as the nerve regenerates.

◆ Nerves regenerate remarkably quickly in the forearm of people of any age and tend to regenerate more quickly in children. The prognosis is best for people under 40, but surgeons do not give up on nerve regeneration in older patients.

◆ No surgeon can guarantee, even with the simplest nerve repair, that normal feeling will come back to the fingertip or other region of the upper limb. Protective sensation can generally be assured, but the finer aspects of touch, such as discriminating texture, cannot always be achieved.

CARPAL TUNNEL SYNDROME

Carpal tunnel syndrome is a common entrapment of an important nerve at the level of the wrist.

A stout fiber ligament overlies the nerve and forms the roof of the carpal tunnel just beyond the wrist crease. Nine flexor tendons keep company with the nerve. These include one flexor tendon to the thumb and two for each of the other fingers. These tendons travel back and forth and are often in forceful use. They press the nerve up against the undersurface of the transverse carpal ligament. Some cases of carpal tunnel

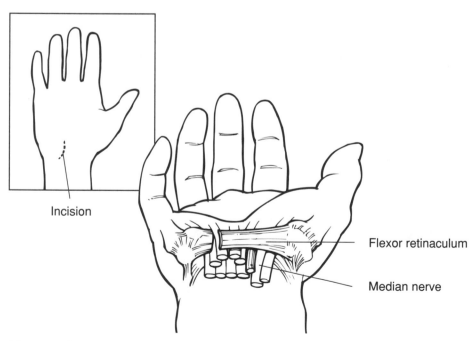

Incision

Flexor retinaculum

Median nerve

Repair of flexor tendons pressing nerve against the carpal ligament

syndrome are the result of repetitive motion at work, but a fair number result simply from ordinary hand use.

People who see their doctor about carpal tunnel syndrome typically complain of numbness and tingling in the thumb, index, middle and half of the ring fingers. This tingling may awaken you from sleep. You may shake your hand as though there is some problem with circulation. Normal feeling returns and you go back to sleep. Such symptoms may come nightly or a few times a week. Sometimes the numbness persists throughout the day and makes you drop objects because of lack of sensory feedback.

In extreme cases, your fingertips may become dry because the nerve fibers that cause sweating on the finger pads are compressed along with the rest of the median nerve. Rarely is there wasting of the thumb wad muscle on the palm of the hand.

Non-Surgical Remedies Surgery is not always necessary to correct the condition.
◆ Varying tasks during work and play may prevent undue pressure on the nerve.
◆ Splinting the wrist at night in a cocked-back position of about 20 degrees reduces the natural tendency to flex the wrist during sleep. The splint keeps your body from pressing on the vulnerable nerve at the wrist.
◆ Anti-inflammatory agents help only if there is also tendinitis or tenosynovitis. An anti-inflammatory agent shrinks the lubricating synovial wrappers on the tendons so the nerve has more room. All anti-inflammatory medicines have side effects, however.
◆ If you are overweight or obese, weight loss is helpful because sometimes nerves are wrapped with fat.
◆ In acute cases, completely stopping for a few weeks whatever activity is causing the problem is helpful.
◆ Injections of steroids by a qualified specialist in the area of the carpal tunnel, well away from the nerve toward the little finger side of the wrist, may be helpful. The steroids shrink the lubricating sleeves on the tendons, allowing more room for the nerve.
◆ If a steroid injection relieves symptoms, even for a few weeks, the prognosis will be very good for an open carpal tunnel release.
◆ If numbness and tingling persist, and in most cases where there has been muscle loss for the numb muscle wad, open carpal tunnel release is recommended.

Surgical Procedure: Open Carpal Tunnel Release This procedure is performed through a small incision that runs from the palm side of the wrist crease out into the near third of the palm. This incision provides an excellent view of the transverse carpal ligament and the carpal tunnel contents, including the nerve and tendons.

If the fiber tissue overlying the tendons at the level of the wrist and the forearm is tight, they can be released through the same incision. Sometimes the incision will be extended farther into the palm and farther up into the forearm.

A carpal tunnel release operation takes 10 to 30 minutes, depending on the complexity of the procedure. Most open carpal tunnel releases are done under local or regional anesthesia. General anesthesia is rarely needed.

In some cases of long-standing sensory motor carpal tunnel syndrome with complete wasting of the thumb muscle wad, a procedure called a tendon transfer, or opponens plasty, is done to restore the thumb's ability to roll over to oppose the other fingers. This tendon transfer adds about 15 or 20 minutes of operating time. The procedure works well.

After the Operation A foam-padded splint is applied to keep the wrist in the cocked-back position (20 degrees extension), with the thumb and fingers free.

◆ Your hand should be elevated above the level of the heart for several days.

◆ The bandage is removed in about one week.

◆ In the second week you will be permitted to move your wrist and hand through a full range of motion, but no power gripping is done.

◆ Sutures are removed at two weeks, and you may gradually return to normal activities over the next four to eight weeks.

◆ If you have had carpal tunnel syndrome symptoms for a year or two, it may take that long to get the full benefit from the procedure. More commonly, the quality of feeling steadily improves over weeks and months.

◆ Muscle tone of the thumb muscle wad will return sometimes partially, sometimes completely. In advanced cases, it may not return at all.

◆ A tendon transfer requires an additional two weeks of immobilization of the wrist and thumb in order to heal.

Surgical Procedure: Endoscopic Carpal Tunnel Release Since the late 1980s, endoscopic carpal tunnel release techniques have been introduced. Extravagant claims have been made about the results. The stated benefits are that the incision is smaller, healing is more rapid and a return to preoperative activity is much faster.

Endoscopic procedures may indeed provide an earlier return to activity, but endoscopic carpal tunnel release remains an experimental treatment.

Consideration of such a technique involves a long discussion with the surgeon, a review of her or his results, including the number of cases done, and a frank discussion of any complications.

◆ One type of endoscopic carpal tunnel release requires an incision measuring about 1 in. (2.5 cm) along the palm side of the wrist crease. An endoscopic blade device is inserted out into the carpal tunnel through this incision so the surgeon can see the undersurface of the ligament. All structures are swept away from the undersurface and the blade is withdrawn toward the wrist crease as the ligament is divided. This is generally done under regional anesthesia, although sometimes it is possible under local anesthesia.

◆ A second type of release is called the two-port approach. This involves an incision at the wrist and a separate incision in the palm, which permits viewing of the ligament from both ends. A blade is used to cut the ligament.

DUPUYTREN'S CONTRACTURE

Dupuytren's contracture is a fibrous thickening of the palm tissue that may feel like nodules or cords. The cords run beneath the skin and feel like firm ridges.

The fiber-supporting structures of the palm skin are called the palmar aponeuroses. This fibrous matrix projects from the near side of the palm all the way out beyond the middle joints of

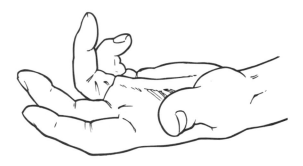

Dupuytren's contracture

the fingers. Myofibroblasts within this fiber matrix have the capacity to contract. As they do, the cords may come together and pull, so that the fingers are curled at the knuckle joints and, in many cases, in the middle joints of the fingers. The ring and little fingers are the most commonly affected.

The main problem of Dupuytren's contracture is functional loss as the fingers draw down into the palm.

This contracture of fiber tissues is most common in people of British Isles descent, western Europeans and Scandinavians. It is five to 10 times more common in men than in women. When women are affected, the process is often accelerated and more severe.

Since the fiber contraction of the palmar aponeuroses may progress a little and then remain stable for many years, there is generally no urgency about surgical intervention for early cases. There is no hard-and-fast rule about when surgery is necessary. It is best to discuss it with an experienced surgeon.

Surgical Procedure Surgery may be done under local anesthesia in simple cases but is usually done under intravenous regional anesthesia because the operation may take up to 90 minutes.

The surgeon makes a zig-zag incision from the near side of the palm out into the fingers, sometimes beyond the middle joints. The cord is carefully and gently separated from nerves, arteries and tendons.

There may not be enough skin to ensure closing the finger in a relaxed position, so sometimes skin grafts are taken from the wrist, elbow or groin. Such skin grafts provide full extension of the finger joints without any tension on the wound edges. These grafts generally heal very nicely.

Occasionally, small areas of incision are left open to heal over by what is called secondary intention. The edges of the skin are separated and the gap closes over a period of one to two weeks. This requires a little more wound care postoperatively.

After the Operation A well-padded dressing with some plaster support is applied, and the wounds are inspected within five or seven days. Sutures are removed at 10 to 14 days.

♦ The hand is gradually remobilized. You should be able to achieve good extension of all joints within four to eight weeks, sometimes longer.

♦ In some cases, a flare response develops. This is an early painful scarring after removal of the Dupuytren's fascia (palmar fasciectomy). It is more common in women than in men and is treated with injections of local anesthesia with or without a steroid mixed with the local.

♦ The recurrence rate after surgical removal of the fibrous cords runs as high as 30 to 40 percent because it is impossible to remove all of the palmar aponeuroses at the time of the operation.

FINGERTIP INJURIES IN CHILDREN

The fingertip is the most commonly injured body part in children, particularly in toddlers, who tend to get their fingers caught in house and car doors. These injuries are terrifying to parents, but they generally heal well.

Surgical Procedure Simple dressings often suffice, and tips that have been partially amputated may be gently repositioned with slender adhesive strips (steri-strips) rather than sutures.

Sometimes several stitches are used to repair subtotal fingertip amputations in toddlers. If a bulky "boxing glove" sterile dressing can be applied even for a few days (challenging in a toddler), very good results are expected.

After the Operation Before age 10, children have a remarkable ability to regenerate fingertips, including nail-forming elements, after injury.

◆ Careful follow-up is required for three to six months, allowing one or two growths of fingernail to occur under observation.

FINGERTIP AMPUTATIONS AND REPLANTATIONS

Amputations in adults present a challenge. With modern microsurgical techniques, it is possible to reattach accidentally amputated parts. This is the province of replantation surgeons schooled in the basic techniques of hand surgery plus microsurgery.

As a general guideline, replantation is appropriate for the tip of the thumb where the amputated part is in good condition and for the loss of two or more digits. Replanting a single digit other than the thumb is usually not done because the remaining fingers can perform most functions.

Replantation is a complex matter that requires careful discussion with the surgeon. People who have amputated parts reattached generally experience some cold intolerance for six to 12 months and sometimes longer. Stiffness is almost inevitable. Repeat operations are necessary in up to half the cases to release scar adhesions of tendon to bone and tendon to tendon sheath. Sometimes repeat operations are necessary for nerve grafting. There may be a period of six months to two years of sophisticated sequential operations to restore function.

Other options require careful and detailed discussion with the surgeon, often with your family included. For example, the most expendable digit in the hand is the index finger, since the middle finger may easily do the index finger's job if the index is completely lost. With thumb loss, some surgeons prefer to transpose the index into the thumb position rather than reattach the thumb.

Surgical Procedure For straightforward fingertip amputations, the surgeon will trim back the tissues to a clean level, permitting the nerve ending to retract into the digit so it is not exposed to trauma. The amputation stump will be gently closed.

Untidy fingertip amputations require a great deal of care, sometimes requiring skin grafts, local flap tissues for coverage or even microsurgical coverage procedures.

Mutilating hand injuries involving multidigit amputations should generally be treated by surgeons who do this type of work all the time.

After the Operation You should have the remainder of the finger back in integrated use with the rest of the hand in a few weeks.

◆ Ninety percent of people whose fingers have been amputated experience "phantom" sensations suggesting that the part is still there. These sensations disappear within six months and are seldom accompanied by pain.

MALLET FINGERS

Mallet or baseball finger is an injury to the thinnest, farthest part of the extensor mechanism that straightens the final joint of the finger. A closed injury such as a jam-type injury from

Mallet finger

playing volleyball or getting hit with a baseball in the fingertip is often enough to tear this paper-thin tendon, causing the fingertip to drop into flexion.

Surgical Procedure Open treatment is seldom necessary, although it may be ideal in some tidy incised wounds of the tendon.

Closed treatment with a splint for eight to 12 weeks is generally sufficient to restore normal extension of the finger, although sometimes there is a 15-degree "lag" in extension.

GANGLION CYSTS

Ganglion cysts often appear as lumps on the top side of the wrist, on the palm side of the wrist (on the thumb side), within the palm or the near side of the finger—feeling like a pebble in the palm—or as small translucent bumps on the top crease of the last joint of the fingers.

The cyst is filled with joint fluid that comes from either the wrist joint or, if the cyst is in the finger or palm or the last joint of the finger, from the flexor sheath. Joint spaces and flexor sheaths are hydraulic systems with fluid under pressure. A small "leak" results in fluid passing from the joint or sheath out into the surrounding tissues. A rather firm lump will be visible under the skin.

These cysts usually do not produce any symptoms. They are benign and are not cancerous.

The treatment of these cysts varies. If you are doing a great deal of repetitive work but can vary your tasks, the cyst will likely go down on its own. Needle aspiration—drawing the fluid out with a syringe—reduces the size of the cyst in 80 or 90 percent of cases, but the cyst will recur. Sometimes patients are successful in "popping" flexor sheath ganglions. Sometimes these ganglions don't come back.

When ganglions come from either the far joint of the finger or the wrist joint, treatment consists of either leaving the cyst alone if it is not troublesome or removing it surgically.

Surgical Procedure Surgical removal with an appropriate anesthetic is curative in 90 percent of cases. In the 10 percent of cases where the cyst comes back, the recurrence is generally due to forceful use too soon after the operation. As a rule, avoid forceful hand and wrist use for about two or three months after surgery.

QUESTIONS TO ASK YOUR HAND SURGEON

◆ What percentage of your practice involves hand surgery?
◆ How many of these operations have you done?
◆ Do you have other patients who would be willing to discuss their experience with this procedure?
◆ How long will my hand be immobilized?
◆ How long will it take to achieve the best result?
◆ How can I help myself to achieve the best possible result?

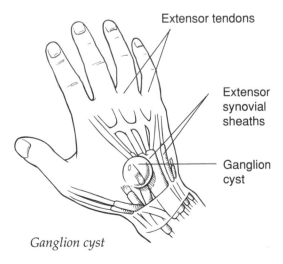

Extensor tendons

Extensor synovial sheaths

Ganglion cyst

Ganglion cyst

17
GYNECOLOGIC SURGERY

Jeanette S. Brown, MD

New techniques, along with improved surgical instruments and anesthetics, have made outpatient surgery a major component of gynecologic care.

Many procedures are now performed using laparoscopy (*see* Chapter 8). In the very near future, with techniques such as laparoscopic assisted vaginal hysterectomy and laparoscopic removal of fibroids, virtually all gynecologic surgeries will be performed either in outpatient surgery centers or with only a one- or two-night stay in the hospital.

THE FEMALE REPRODUCTIVE SYSTEM

Knowledge of pelvic anatomy and terminology is important for a complete understanding of gynecologic surgery.

The uterus (womb), the fallopian tubes and the ovaries are in the lower abdomen. The uterus is about the size of a person's fist. The fallopian tubes are even narrower than a pencil. The ovaries are the size of walnuts. Although the tubes and ovaries are close together, they are not connected.

Above the uterus and vagina is the bladder, where urine is collected. From it leads the urethra, the tube through which urine is passed out of the body. The rectum, for the passage of stool, is behind the vagina and uterus.

The cervix is the part of the uterus in the vagina that can be seen during a pelvic exam. The opening into the uterine cavity is called the cervical os.

The lining of the uterus, or endometrium, is what is shed each month during the menstrual cycle.

COMMON DANGER SIGNS AFTER SURGERY

The specifics of your medical care, both before and after an operation, should be discussed extensively with your gynecologist. But you should be aware of common postoperative danger signs. If any one of these symptoms appears after your procedure, contact your gynecologist immediately.

◆ A temperature greater than 100.4°F (38°C).

◆ Heavy vaginal bleeding such as soaking a sanitary napkin every one to two hours.

◆ Severe lower abdominal cramping or pain.

◆ Dizziness, fainting or weakness.

ABNORMAL UTERINE BLEEDING: DILATATION AND CURETTAGE (D&C) AND OTHER PROCEDURES

Abnormal uterine bleeding occurs most often in the teenage years and when menopause is occurring. There are several common causes of abnormal uterine bleeding, including miscarriage,

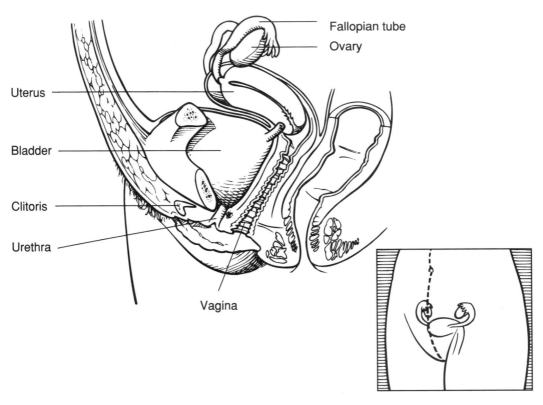

Female reproductive system

cancer, cervical or endometrial polyps, fibroids and cancer.

♦ Cancer is uncommon in younger women. In women over 35, however, cancer of the lining of the uterus must be considered whenever there is abnormal bleeding.

♦ Cervical polyps are benign growths of the lining of the cervix. The polyp is seen protruding from the cervical os and may be removed in the office.

♦ An endometrial polyp is a benign growth of the lining of the uterus and cannot be seen during a pelvic exam.

♦ Fibroids are benign growths in the muscle of the uterus. Abnormal bleeding often occurs if the fibroids are near the endometrium.

When abnormal bleeding occurs, a biopsy of the uterine lining (endometri-al biopsy) may be done in the office using a small, thin catheter. If the bleeding has been heavy, a slightly larger catheter is attached to a suction machine to remove more of the endometrium.

Dilatation and Curettage Often referred to as a D&C, this is one of the most common gynecologic outpatient procedures. It is performed to diagnose the cause of abnormal uterine bleeding, including bleeding in postmenopausal women. A D&C is rarely required in younger women because cancer is so uncommon in women under 35.

A D&C is often an office procedure, but it may be performed in an outpatient surgery center for a number of reasons. At times, the gynecologist is unable to enter the endometrial cavity through the cervical os because of cervical scarring (stenosis). In some cases, the office procedure may be too painful for the patient. Or there may be either insufficient tissue to confirm a diagnosis or continued heavy bleeding after the office sampling.

The operation is usually performed under regional or general anesthesia.

Surgical Procedure The surgeon gently opens the cervix with graduated dilators. This allows for the passage of a sharp curved curet into the uterus to remove the endometrial lining. The curet is passed a number of times to ensure that all areas of the endometrium are sampled and removed.

The D&C is both diagnostic and therapeutic. The cause of the bleeding is determined. The bleeding is stopped by the removal of polyps or excess endometrium.

Hysteroscopy If bleeding continues after the D&C or the cause of the abnormal bleeding remains unclear, a hysteroscopy to view the uterine cavity is recommended.

This is done in the office or in an outpatient surgery center. The cervix is dilated so a small scope can pass through the os to view the uterine cavity. Most often a small endometrial polyp or a fibroid missed on the D&C is seen protruding into the endometrial cavity.

The hysteroscope may also be used to perform operative procedures in the uterine cavity. Small scissors or a laser may be passed through the hysteroscope

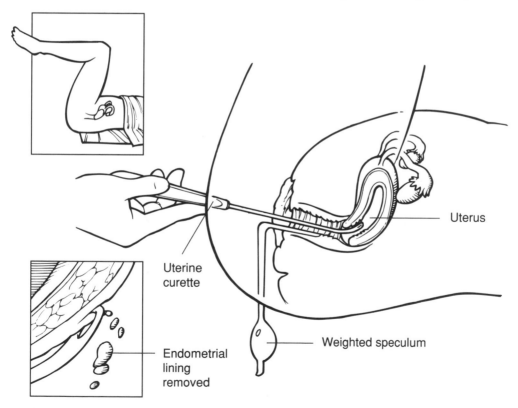

Uterus

Uterine curette

Endometrial lining removed

Weighted speculum

Dilatation and Curettage

to remove a uterine septum or to cut scarring of the uterine lining (Asherman's syndrome).

Endometrial Ablation This new procedure may be considered for women who continue to bleed despite all therapies and who do not desire future fertility. A "roller-ball" instrument is used through the hysteroscope to burn (coagulate) the endometrial lining. After the procedure, patients will no longer have any bleeding, although a small number may continue with spotting.

After the Operation During the D&C or hysteroscopy, there is a small risk of perforating the uterus. If this occurs, the uterus often heals on its own, and additional surgery is rarely needed.
◆ You may usually resume your normal activities within one day of the operation.
◆ Irregular spotting, light bleeding and slight to moderate pelvic discomfort and cramping are expected for one to two weeks.
◆ Intercourse should not be resumed for two weeks.

CONE BIOPSY

The Pap (Papanicolaou) smear is a screening test for precancer and cancer of the cervix. An abnormal Pap smear showing a precancerous condition called dysplasia/cervical intraepithelial neoplasia requires a follow-up office procedure called a colposcopy. The colposcope is an instrument that magnifies the cervix so the gynecologist can identify and biopsy abnormal areas.

When the colposcopic biopsy confirms a small precancerous condition, an office procedure to remove the abnormal lesions is done with either a freezing of the cervix (cryosurgery) or a laser.

A cone biopsy is recommended if the office procedure has failed, abnormal areas are large and extend high into the cervical os or there is a possibility of a cervical cancer.

Surgical Procedure During a cone biopsy, the abnormal area on the cervix is removed as a small cone of cervical tissue with a scalpel or laser. The tissue is then examined to confirm the diagnosis of a precancerous condition and ensure that there is no cancer. Most often the cone biopsy is also sufficient treatment of the precancerous condition.

In very rare cases, women may have difficulty becoming pregnant or may have early labor after a cone biopsy.

After the Operation You will probably be able to resume your normal activities in two or three days.
◆ Irregular spotting, light bleeding and slight pelvic discomfort are expected for one to two weeks.
◆ Intercourse should not be resumed for at least one month and then only after your gynecologist's approval.

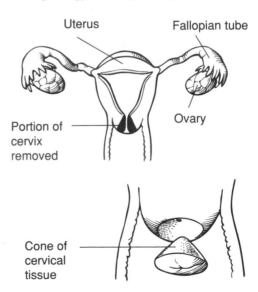

Cone biopsy

◆ Heavy bleeding that soaks one sanitary napkin every one to two hours may occur, usually seven to 10 days after surgery. Contact your gynecologist immediately if there is heavy bleeding.

LAPAROSCOPY

For years, laparoscopy has been used extensively in gynecology to view the pelvic organs to diagnose the cause of pelvic pain, infertility and ectopic pregnancy. Recently, operative laparoscopy using operating instruments and a laser has allowed surgeons to treat these problems.

Surgical Procedure For the laparoscopic procedure, you will be placed in the Trendelenburg position, in which you are tilted at a 45-degree angle, with your head and shoulders pointing toward the floor. This helps keep the bowel out of the operative field.

At the beginning of any laparoscopic procedure, a small incision is made just below the navel. A needle-like instrument is passed into the abdominal cavity to fill the abdomen with carbon dioxide gas. The gas creates a clear pocket to safely pass the larger laparoscope.

Another small incision is made above the pubic bone, through which operating instruments are inserted. Depending on the type of laparoscopic surgery to be performed, additional instruments may be inserted in each side of the abdomen.

There are some risks involved in laparoscopic surgery, some of the most serious occurring during the placement of the instruments through the abdomen. Injury to the bowel or bladder is possible. Hemorrhaging may occur with instrument placement or during the operative procedure.

After the Operation Depending on the extent of the laparoscopic surgery, most women may resume their normal activities within seven days.

◆ It is common to have some shoulder pain after being in the Trendelenburg position and to have irritation from the gas in the abdomen.

◆ Mild to moderate incisional and abdominal pain is expected for one to two weeks.

◆ Intercourse should not be resumed for two weeks.

STERILIZATION THROUGH TUBAL LIGATION

This is one of the oldest and most common procedures performed with the laparoscope. Tubal ligation—sometimes referred to as "having your tubes tied"—is the most effective form of contraception, with a failure rate of less than 1 percent. Sterilization is permanent, so you must be clear about not wanting future fertility.

Male sterilization with a vasectomy is less expensive and safer than laparoscopic tubal ligation and should be considered. It should also be noted that spousal consent is not legally required to have sterilization.

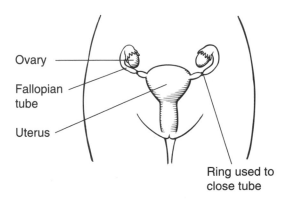

Ovary

Fallopian tube

Uterus

Ring used to close tube

Tubal ligation

147

Surgical Procedure An instrument is passed through the lower abdominal incision. The fallopian tube may be sealed by coagulation or by placing a small plastic ring to strangulate the tube. Both techniques block the passage of sperm and ova (eggs) along the tube.

After the Operation Failures may occur after sterilization, although they are rare (about one in every 250 procedures).
◆ If you suspect a pregnancy at any time after sterilization, contact your gynecologist immediately. As many as 50 percent of pregnancies after sterilization are ectopic pregnancies. (*See* "Ectopic Pregnancy" at the end of this chapter.)

DIAGNOSTIC LAPAROSCOPY FOR CHRONIC PELVIC PAIN

Chronic pelvic pain is caused by many diseases, the most common being endometriosis and prior pelvic inflammatory disease (PID). Both may cause scar tissue to form in the pelvis, which may also contribute to pelvic pain.
◆ Endometriosis is the term used to describe implants of endometrial tissue outside the uterus. These implants may be found throughout the pelvic area and they respond to hormonal cycles similiar to the lining of the uterus. Most women with endometriosis have very painful menstrual cycles.
◆ PID is caused by infectious organisms—the most common are gonorrhea and chlamydia—that ascend into the uterus, tubes or ovaries. The infection may cause tubal damage, abscesses and scars.

Surgical Procedure At the time of diagnostic laparoscopy for endometriosis, electrocauterization or a laser is used to remove the implants, as well as any scar tissue and ovarian cysts (endometriomas).

In the case of PID, during laparoscopy the scar tissue may be removed and blocked tubes may be opened to decrease the chronic pain.

LAPAROSCOPIC TREATMENT FOR INFERTILITY

Laparoscopy is often used to discover the cause of infertility. If either endometriosis or indications of prior PID are found, similiar procedures as outlined above are followed.

The gynecologist may also confirm that the fallopian tubes are open by pushing dye through the uterus while observing if it flows out the ends of both tubes.

The newer techniques for treatment of infertility are:
◆ in vitro fertilization (IVF);
◆ gamete intrafallopian tube transfer (GIFT); and
◆ zygote intrafallopian tube transfer (ZIFT).

Procedure: IVF This is usually performed as an office procedure for women whose fallopian tubes are blocked.

Ultrasound imaging is used to locate the maturing eggs (ova) in the ovaries. The ova are collected from the ovaries with a small needle passed through the vagina. In the laboratory, the ova are mixed with sperm and fertilized. These embryos are then placed in the uterus .

Surgical Procedure: GIFT and ZIFT For women with normal fallopian tubes, GIFT and ZIFT are performed laparoscopically. In both procedures, the ova are collected from the ovaries through the laparoscope.
◆ With GIFT, the collected ova and sperm are placed in the fallopian tube.
◆ ZIFT is similiar to IVF. The collected

ova are mixed with sperm in the laboratory, and the resulting embryos are placed in the fallopian tube.

REMOVING OVARIAN CYSTS AND OVARIES

The ovary produces many types of benign cysts and it is not always necessary to remove them. But an ovarian cyst should be removed when it is persistent, lasts more than a few months, continues to increase in size or causes pain.

Surgical Procedure In a procedure called a cystectomy, the cyst is removed by carefully separating it from the ovary. The cyst is then examined to ensure that it is benign.

In rare instances, the cyst cannot be separated from the ovary, in which case the ovary must be removed as well (oophorectomy).

ECTOPIC PREGNANCY

An ectopic pregnancy occurs when a fertilized egg (ovum) becomes implanted somewhere other than in the uterus.

Most commonly, an ectopic pregnancy occurs midway along the fallopian tube and is often called a tubal pregnancy. The placenta invades the tube and eventually can cause the tube to rupture. A tubal rupture may lead to life-threatening internal bleeding.

An ectopic pregnancy must be removed. It may be possible to avoid surgery through a new approach that involves using methotrexate, a chemotherapy drug. Once the diagnosis of ectopic pregnancy has been made, the patient is given one shot of the methotrexate, which destroys the cells of the pregnancy.

Surgical Procedure Either a laser or laparoscopic scissors open the tube over the ectopic pregnancy. The pregnancy is removed with suction. The fallopian tube will heal on its own.

After the Operation Persistent ectopic pregnancies have been reported with both laparoscopic and methotrexate treatments, so it is essential to have close follow-up after these procedures.

QUESTIONS TO ASK YOUR GYNECOLOGIST
◆ How much bleeding should I expect after the procedure?
◆ When may I resume my normal activities?
◆ When may I resume sexual relations?

18
UROLOGIC SURGERY

Marshall L. Stoller, MD, and Damien Bolton, MD

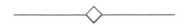

Urology is the field of surgery concerned with the urinary system and the organs of the male reproductive tract.

Several surgical procedures to the scrotum and penis are commonly performed on an outpatient basis. Surgery to the urinary system often involves a hospital stay, although many diagnostic examinations and the non-invasive treatment of kidney stones are routinely performed as outpatient procedures.

More extensive outpatient surgery of the urinary tract may be possible in the future with the continuing development of laparoscopic urologic techniques (*see also* Chapter 8).

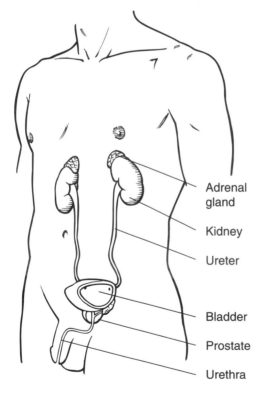

Adrenal gland

Kidney

Ureter

Bladder

Prostate

Urethra

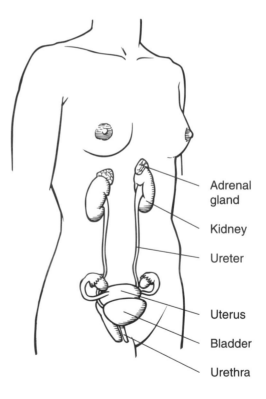

Adrenal gland

Kidney

Ureter

Uterus

Bladder

Urethra

Male and female urinary tract

THE URINARY SYSTEM AND THE MALE REPRODUCTIVE TRACT

The kidneys lie next to the spinal cord against the back wall of the abdomen. Kidneys have the job of filtering our blood as well as regulating the balance of water and salt and the acidity of body fluids. Each kidney has about a million small filters called nephrons, and as blood passes through these nephrons, urine is produced and collected.

The ureters are narrow, muscular tubes that carry the urine from the kidneys to the bladder for storage. When the bladder is full, the urine is discharged through the urethra, a tube about 2 in. (5 cm) long in women and about four times as long in men. The urinary sphincter is the muscle, normally contracted, that maintains continence and regulates the urinary flow.

In males, the urethra also carries secretions from the prostate, a walnut-sized gland surrounding the urethra where it leaves the bladder, as well as secretions from the seminal vesicles and sperm from the vas deferens.

DIAGNOSTIC PROCEDURES

For a thorough evaluation of the urinary tract, a number of diagnostic and treatment techniques are routinely combined. The most common outpatient procedure, cystoscopy, is often combined with retrograde pyelography or bladder biopsy.

Procedure: Cystoscopy This procedure takes 15 to 20 minutes. It is designed to collect information about the diameter of the urethra, the size and obstructing potential of the prostate, the reason for

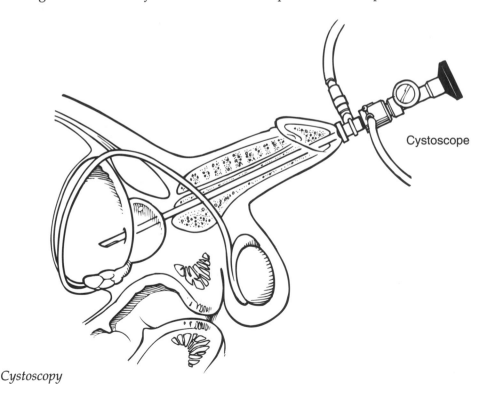

Cystoscopy

recent infections and the cause of blood loss from the urinary tract.

Cystoscopy has traditionally been performed under local anesthesia using a rigid telescope. More recently, smaller and more flexible instruments have been used. If your urologist plans to perform the cystoscopy under anything other than local anesthesia, you will have to abstain from eating and drinking after midnight the night before.

A local anesthetic gel is injected into the genital area in a female or at the end of the penis in a male. A telescope is then inserted through the urethra into the bladder to permit inspection of the bladder and its associated structures.

After the Procedure For a day or two after the cystoscopy, you may experience some burning and stinging when passing urine and you may feel the need to pass urine more frequently. You also may notice small amounts of blood in the urine. This is normal.

Other symptoms might develop if the cystoscopy was combined with other procedures.

Surgical Procedure: Bladder Biopsy If a bladder abnormality is visible on cystoscopy, the urologist will use a special instrument to remove a small piece of tissue for pathology lab analysis to find the cause.

After the Operation Bleeding from the bladder wall is usual after a biopsy. This will be minimized by cauterizing the affected area, but it is normal to have small amounts of blood in the urine for several days. If you have significant bleeding, with large clots in the urine and difficulty in urinating, however, contact your urologist immediately.

Surgical Procedure: Testes Biopsy A biopsy of the testes may be done as part of an investigation of male infertility.

The tissue sample is taken through an incision in the scrotum.

After the Operation As with all scrotal surgery, rest and recuperation are necessary afterwards to prevent bleeding, and pain relief medications will have to be provided.

Diagnostic Laparoscopy In diagnostic laparoscopy, the pelvis and abdomen are examined using an intra-abdominal camera. This may help identify the cause of pelvic pain or determine tumor spread in prostate or bladder cancers.

The lymph nodes from the abdomen or pelvis may be sampled at the same time to confirm or exclude tumor spread, but this procedure requires three or four small incisions in the abdominal wall and is rarely performed on an outpatient basis.

X-Ray Studies Your urologist may order a range of diagnostic radiological studies. These all involve instilling contrast dye through a catheter in an attempt to identify abnormalities in the bladder or urethra. Several x-rays may be taken during these procedures, so it is important that you inform your urologist ahead of time if there is any possibility that you might be pregnant.

◆ With a vasogram, the x-ray contrast dye is injected into the vas deferens to indicate any obstructions between the testes and the urinary tract.

◆ With a cystogram, the bladder alone is viewed.

◆ A urethrogram produces an image of the urethra.

◆ With a voiding cystourethrogram, attention is paid to the reflux of urine back up the ureter and into the kidney when the contrast is voided out of the bladder. Significant amounts of reflux may indicate the cause of recurrent kidney infections or other urinary tract conditions. Antibiotic therapy or even

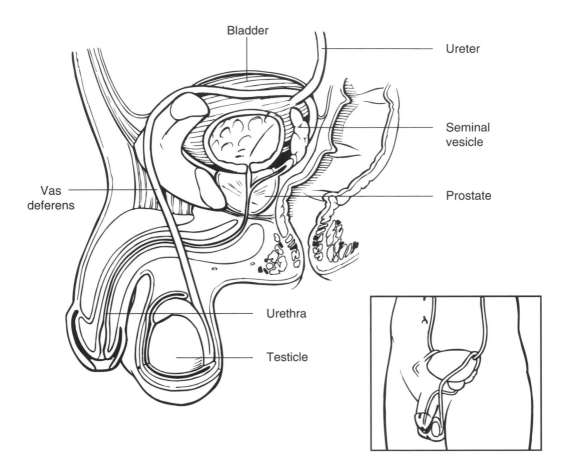

Cross-section of male genitourinary tract

surgical correction by reimplanting the ureter in another site within the bladder wall may be necessary.

◆ Occasionally, the same x-ray contrast dye is injected through the tip of the penis to outline the urethra in its course from the penis to the bladder. This is done to find any narrowing or blockages within the urethra or to investigate urinary incontinence. During this procedure, a clamp may be placed on the outside of the penis or a balloon catheter may be placed within the end of the urethra to permit the contrast dye to fully outline the urethra.

You will not need an anesthetic for any of these procedures.

Procedure: Retrograde Pyelography A retrograde pyelogram is performed when routine x-rays do not show the ureter clearly enough.

A small catheter is placed through the bladder into the opening of the ureter and an x-ray-visible contrast dye is injected into the ureter to outline its course from the bladder to the kidney.

If any abnormalities are found, a syringe may be attached to the catheter and samples of urine taken from the ureter and kidney on the affected side. A laboratory analysis of the samples may reveal evidence of tumors, recent infections or other conditions.

Ultrasound Examinations Ultrasound involves emitting high-frequency sound waves from a probe placed on the skin. The waves are reflected in varying intensities to produce an image of an organ on a video screen.

Ultrasound evaluation of some or all parts of the urinary tract are normally performed as outpatient procedures, the most common being assessments of the kidneys (renal ultrasound) and the prostate gland (transrectal ultrasound).

◆ *Kidney.* Renal ultrasound may allow kidney abnormalities to be identified and may provide enough information to eliminate the need for an intravenous pyelogram. The ultrasound has the advantage of eliminating radiation exposure. The procedure is painless and non-invasive.

To get a superior image, the ultrasonographer will place a cold gel on your skin through which the sound waves from the probe can be better transmitted. You may also be asked to move about on the examination table to get the best image.

◆ *Prostate Gland.* This is often performed in combination with a biopsy to exclude or confirm the presence of cancer in the prostate. You will usually be required to fast from midnight the night before the procedure.

You will have to have an enema to evacuate your bowels. You will also be given antibiotics to reduce the small risk of infection, so you should notify your urologist of any antibiotic sensitivities or allergies.

An ultrasound probe, slightly wider than a finger, will be inserted into the rectum to obtain a close-up image of the prostate. Regions that appear abnormal may suggest sites of cancer, and these may be biopsied at the same time.

The biopsies are performed using a spring-loaded needle, which is inserted into the gland under guidance provided by the ultrasound machine. Such needles fire automatically at a rapid speed, which is uncomfortable but not usually painful. A small core of prostate tissue is taken, which is sent to a pathologist for examination.

After the Procedure Discomfort in the groin and between your legs may last for up to 24 hours.

◆ You will have some blood in both your urine and stools for two or three days. This bleeding is caused by the biopsy needle and is normal. Should the bleeding become heavy, with the passage of large clots, or if you have difficulty passing urine, contact your urologist immediately.

◆ Also notify your urologist immediately if you develop a high fever, chills or night sweats. Infection is the major risk of this procedure, although it is uncommon.

Urodynamic Studies A urodynamic profile evaluates the pressures produced in the bladder and in the urinary sphincter during voiding and at various levels of bladder filling.

The profile documents the bladder's ability to contract and empty urine to completion, the likelihood of uncontrolled or unstable contractions that may produce incontinence and the degree to which the urinary sphincter is functioning.

Multiple tracings are made on recording paper as the bladder is filled to provide a record of the pressures achieved after various volumes of water or gas have been pumped in. The recordings provide excellent insights into the functioning of the bladder, and thereby also into the causes and appropriate treatments for conditions affecting the lower genito-urinary tract.

A urodynamic study is best performed while you are awake so you can tell the urologist when your bladder feels full and when you first feel the need to void. The study lasts between 45 and 60 minutes and is not painful. ·

A local anesthetic gel is placed in the urethra to numb the region, then a small catheter is passed into the bladder. Sterile water, or in some cases gas, is slowly pumped into the bladder until it is full. The pressures in the bladder are recorded with the catheter.

Another catheter may be placed in the rectum to measure the intra-abdominal pressure. This allows the precise measurement of the pressures generated when the bladder contracts. Both catheters are kept in place by taping them to the thigh.

◆ If the urodynamic study is being done to identify or evaluate urinary stress incontinence—where incontinence is initiated or made worse by coughing, sneezing or straining—your urologist may ask you to stand or sit during the procedure to document bladder pressures in various postures.

◆ At the end of the procedure, the catheters will be gently and painlessly pulled out of the bladder and rectum.

After the Procedure The catheter may irritate the urethra's lining, so you may note some burning or stinging while urinating. These symptoms subside without treatment over the first 24 hours. If they persist or if symptoms of infection develop—fevers, sweats and loin pain—notify your urologist.

Depending on the nature of the recordings, your urologist may be able to discuss the results with you immediately. It is far more likely, however, that it will take time to examine them in detail, so a follow-up visit will be arranged.

DRAINING THE BLADDER AND KIDNEYS

Your urologist may leave one or more catheters in place after a urologic procedure. These prevent urinary leakage and permit complete evacuation of urine from the kidney or bladder.

With all forms of catheter drainage of the urinary tract, there will be irritation of the collecting system of the kidney or bladder. Bacteria will also colonize the urine, so bacteriologic cultures from such tubes will always be positive, but this is of no concern unless the tubes become obstructed.

Draining the Bladder The Foley bladder catheter is the most commonly used. It is made of either latex rubber or silicone plastic, so irritation to the lining of the urinary tract is minimal.

◆ The catheter is a long, thin tube of varying width held within the bladder by an inflatable balloon. The balloon pulls against the neck of the bladder and/or the prostate gland to prevent the catheter from falling out. The balloon is inflated with water through a side port. A built-in valve ensures that it stays inflated. The catheter drains through several small holes in its tip beyond the balloon, down through the catheter and into a urine bag connected to the external opening.

◆ Normal handling will not cause the catheter to fall out or become dislodged.

◆ After leaving the hospital, you will most probably use a bag that is attached to the side of your leg by Velcro fasteners. This leg bag may be emptied into the toilet or any other receptacle by pulling down on a device at the bottom of the bag. This device must be firmly clipped in the closed position after emptying to prevent leakage.

◆ Because the Foley catheter may be left in place for some time, good hygiene is

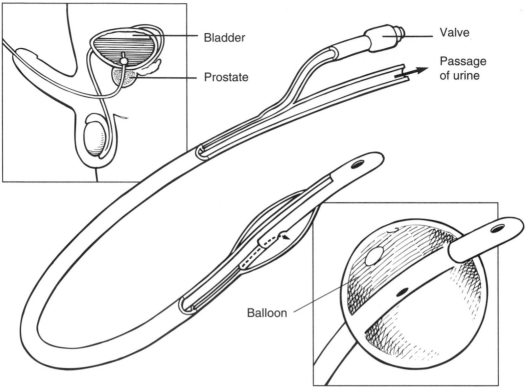

Bladder

Prostate

Valve

Passage of urine

Balloon

Foley bladder catheter

essential to prevent the opening of the urethra from becoming inflamed. No harm will come from washing around the catheter with water or by bathing, but be careful not to pull hard on the catheter while the balloon is inflated because it may cause pain and bleeding from the urethra.

♦ You may have some discomfort in the urinary tract and feel the need to urinate frequently while the catheter is in place. This is normal, but call your doctor if these symptoms become severe or if other complications such as bleeding develop.

♦ Your urologist will remove the catheter painlessly after deflating the balloon with an empty syringe.

Suprapubic Catheter (Cystostomy) This type of catheter is used to relieve the

bladder of urine without having a catheter pass through the urethra.

♦ It usually enters the bladder about 1 in. (2.5 cm) above the pubic bone and is connected to a standard catheter bag. These catheters are of the Foley balloon type or they are kept in place either by multiple arms, or flanges, or occasionally by being sutured to the wall of the abdomen.

♦ A dressing around the exit site keeps the region clean and secures the catheter against accidental removal.

♦ Even with such a catheter, you may still feel the need to void and may occasionally even pass a significant amount of urine through the urethra. If your suprapubic catheter is not draining at all, however, or if you have symptoms such as pain, fever or bleeding, call your urologist.

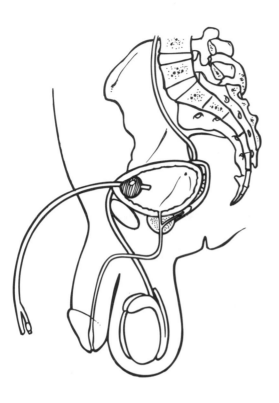

Suprapubic catheter (cystostomy)

Draining the Kidney A nephrostomy tube may be inserted to relieve a kidney obstruction due to a blockage of the ureter or as part of the plan to manage kidney stones or infections.

◆ You will be given a local anesthesia such as lidocaine injected into the back. A needle is directed through the skin and down into the collecting system of the kidney. A wire is then passed through the needle into the collecting system, permitting the passage of larger and larger dilators and, eventually, the nephrostomy tube itself.

◆ The tube is secured by stitching it to the skin of the back, then taping it in place. The tube is fixed within the kidney's collecting system with an attached string that can be pulled to twist the tube into a tight loop.

◆ A nephrostomy tube will drain urine from the kidney on the side on which it was placed, but will not drain urine from the other kidney. If a double-J stent is in place on the same side as the nephrostomy tube, urine from the opposite kidney may occasionally reflux up from the bladder through the stent and into the collecting system, then drain out through the nephrostomy tube.

◆ The nephrostomy tube is usually connected to a drainage system similar to that used for a Foley bladder catheter, namely leg bags.

◆ As with any urinary catheter, a nephrostomy tube will irritate the lining of the collecting system, so you may see blood in your urine. This is not a major concern unless there is a lot of blood or it contains clots.

◆ There will always be some redness at the tube insertion site.

Caring for the Nephrostomy Tube The care of your nephrostomy tube is a complicated and detailed matter, and you should not hesitate to call your urologist if you feel there are any problems.

◆ Contact your urologist immediately if the tube doesn't seem to be draining urine adequately, if there is excessive pain or blood loss through or around the tube or if you develop a high fever, nausea or vomiting.

◆ It is important to exercise the greatest caution at all times when moving or redressing nephrostomy tubes to prevent them from accidentally being pulled from the kidney.

◆ Care should be taken to prevent the tubes from kinking. Kinking impedes drainage and leads to a build-up of urine in the kidney, which may cause infection.

◆ Long-term nephrostomy tubes have to be changed every three to four months and need special attention at all times to permit adequate drainage.

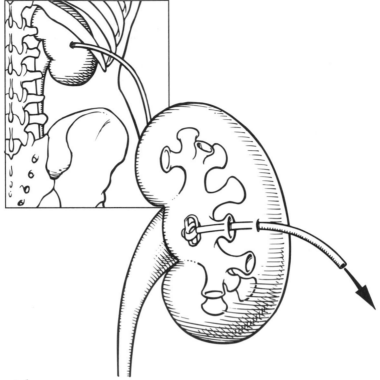

Nephrostomy tube

◆ Blockages may develop in a securely dressed and non-kinked system because of small blood clots or other solid matter in the tube. Your urologist or nurse will usually be able to help by flushing the tube with a sterile saline solution or vacuuming out the offending material. Significant infections may result from this procedure, so it should never be done by anyone other than trained medical staff. Antibiotics and the drawing of urine specimens for analysis may be required, and secure redressing of the drainage system is always essential.

◆ A nephrostomy tube may be left in place to drain one or both kidneys either instead of, or in addition to, a Foley catheter draining the bladder. These catheters enter the skin underneath the ribs and pass into the collect-ing system of the kidney, which is then able to drain into bags attached to the catheters.

◆ After you are discharged from the hospital, the catheter bags may be exchanged for leg bags.

◆ You will be able to bath or shower with a nephrostomy tube in place.

After the Tubes Are Removed
Discomfort and blood in the urine may persist for several days after a drainage tube is removed.

◆ Under normal circumstances, these symptoms will subside within 48 hours. If they become excessive, call your treating physician immediately.

◆ Normal activities should be resumed gradually, otherwise you may have recurrent bleeding, especially after having a nephrostomy catheter removed.

TREATING URINARY STONES

Urinary stones, or calculi, occur more often in men than in women. They form in the collecting system of the kidney and may grow to a size of several inches. More commonly, they migrate down the ureter when they are still very small. If the stone is longer than 1/4 in. (5 mm), it is too large to pass through the urinary tract on its own, so it will require surgical treatment.

Until about 10 years ago, treatment usually involved open surgery. An incision was made in the muscles of the abdomen and the surgeon cut down into the kidney or ureter, found the stone and removed it. With the development of sophisticated instruments during the 1980s, however, particularly those using fiberoptic lenses or shock waves, stones are now treated without an incision and largely as an outpatient procedure.

Before the Operation You may have to undergo one or more x-ray examinations before treatment, the most common being an intravenous pyelogram, or IVP. This involves taking a series of x-ray pictures before and after a contrast dye is injected into the bloodstream.

An IVP helps determine the number and size of the stones as well as their position in the urinary collecting system.

You will have to take laxatives to clear the bowel before the IVP so that a better image of the kidneys is obtained.

The dye is injected usually into a vein in the forearm. You may feel a warmth somewhat like a hot flush and may also notice a metallic taste in your

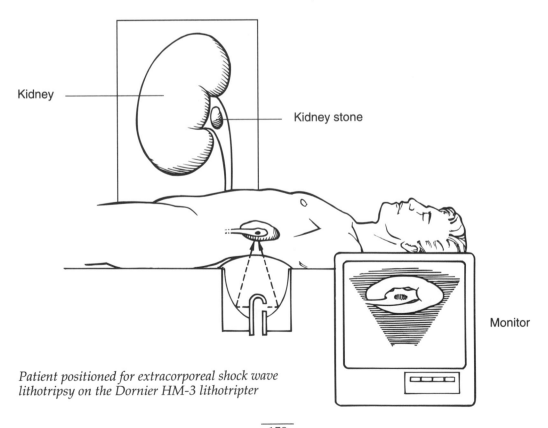

Kidney

Kidney stone

Monitor

Patient positioned for extracorporeal shock wave lithotripsy on the Dornier HM-3 lithotripter

mouth. Allergic reactions to the dye are uncommon and other complications are rare. The procedure usually takes about 45 minutes.

Surgical Procedure: Extracorporeal Shock Wave Lithotripsy In the 10 years since the procedure was introduced, extracorporeal shock wave lithotripsy, or ESWL, has become a standard treatment for most stones in the kidney and the upper ureter. More than a million patients have now been treated by this generally safe and effective method of fragmenting stones without an incision.

Ultrasound or x-rays are used to locate the stones, and shock waves from an external source pass through the body wall and are focused at those points. The stones fragment into many pieces about the size of grains of sand. These are then passed in the urine—with minimal if any pain—over the next few weeks.

ESWL is usually done either with sedation alone or with a spinal anesthetic, although a general anesthetic may be required, particularly if the stone has to be pushed from the ureter into the kidney so it can be seen and treated more easily.

The form of lithotripsy you experience will depend on which lithotripsy device is used. With older machines, patients sit in a waterbath so the shock waves pass into the body without having to go through air, which may reduce their effect. With newer machines, the shock waves pass through a water cushion.

During treatment, you may notice ever greater degrees of discomfort with the gradual increase in power. Low-voltage waves may feel like a small pin prick. More intense waves will require more complete anesthesia.

How many shock waves will be applied depends on many factors, including the size of the stone, its posi-

tion in the urinary tract, how long you've had it and the energy level of the shock wave used. For most stones, the standard treatment ranges between 2,000 and 6,000 shock waves, which can be administered in 45 minutes to just over an hour.

Inserting a Stent If your stone is so large that the fragments might block the urinary tract when passed, your urologist may place a tube, or stent, from the bladder to the kidney during the lithotripsy procedure. The stent has a curling loop in the kidney and another in the bladder to prevent it from shifting up or down in the urinary tract. It is called a double-J stent because of its shape.

Although it may cause some bladder discomfort and some blood in the urine afterwards, the stent plays an important part in making sure the kidney continues to drain.

The stent is removed under a local anesthetic and without significant discomfort. It may be placed with an attached string protruding through the urethra, in which case the stent is removed in your doctor's office simply by pulling the string. This should be done only by, or on the specific instructions of, your urologist.

After the ESWL Treatment You can expect to spend one to two hours recovering from the anesthesia before being discharged home, usually the same day.
◆ You will pass numerous stone fragments during the first few weeks, usually with no pain or discomfort. Your urologist may ask you to urinate through a square of gauze or some other type of strainer to collect some fragments for analysis.
◆ Most stones will pass through the urinary tract within the first six weeks, but small fragments often remain in the kidney or ureter for up to three months.

Your urologist will usually order a repeat x-ray around this time to make sure all the fragments have passed.

◆ In the vast majority of cases, ESWL is performed without any significant complications.

◆ You may notice blood in your urine. There will be more blood if you have a double-J stent, and this may persist for as long as the stent is left inside.

◆ You may feel some pain on the side treated by lithotripsy, although this is usually mild and is managed with oral analgesics such as Tylenol.

◆ Occasionally, a bruise or abrasion appears at the point on the back over the kidney where the shock waves entered the body. This usually clears up within a few days, and oral analgesics take care of any discomfort.

◆ Rarely, more serious complications develop. If there was a significant infection in the kidney at the time of treatment, a fever may result from bacteria spreading through the bloodstream. This might be accompanied by nausea and vomiting. If these symptoms appear, contact your urologist immediately. You may have to be admitted to the hospital for antibiotic therapy.

◆ Stone fragments occasionally obstruct the ureter, causing pain, sometimes severe, as well as nausea, vomiting or fever. This usually happens when large stones are treated by ESWL. In rare cases, a blockage occurs despite having a double-J stent inserted to prevent it. Contact your urologist immediately if you develop these symptoms.

The Need for Retreatment How many ESWL treatments you need depends mainly on the type and size of your stones. If they are very large, two or three sessions may be planned to make sure they are all cleared, but a single session is usually enough for most people.

Those who are more likely to need a second treatment include people who are heavier than the normal range for their height, those in whom the stones are poorly seen on x-rays and those who have stones in a peripheral part of the urinary collecting system that might be partially blocked or poorly drained.

The type of machine used is also a factor, although the rate at which additional treatment is required tends to be fairly constant — 10 to 20 percent of cases.

Additional treatments may be necessary even after complete fragmentation if stones reform. This may happen for a variety of reasons, including a failure to drink enough water and other fluids, an excess of a particular substance in the diet or an inborn tendency to make stones of a particular chemical type.

To help prevent future stones, your urologist will usually have you collect urine for 24 hours and arrange blood tests and stone analysis to discover why the stones formed in the first place. Stone analysis helps determine the type of stone and may also indicate dietary changes or medications that could reduce the likelihood of your making more stones.

If no steps are taken to reduce the rate of stone formation, about 50 percent of patients develop new stones over five years.

Surgical Procedure: Ureteroscopy
ESWL is the standard treatment for most stones in the kidney and the upper urinary tract. Stones in the lower third of the ureter are usually treated by ureteroscopy.

No skin incision is involved, but anesthesia is necessary, usually the same form as for ESWL. Ureteroscopy is usually performed in the modified lithotomy position, meaning that you will lie on your back with your legs elevated in stirrups.

A telescope is inserted into the bladder through the urethra and is advanced into the ureter until the stone can be seen. Most ureteroscopes are long, rigid instruments through which the tools needed to fragment and remove the stones are easily passed. Occasionally, a flexible ureteroscope is used.

Your urologist may also use a high-pressure balloon to dilate the opening of the ureter as it enters the bladder. This will ease the passage of the ureteroscope and make it easier to extract large stones or fragments.

The stones are collected in specially designed baskets or are grasped by instruments and removed intact. If the stone is too large to be removed unbroken, it may be fragmented by ultrasound, lasers, electrohydraulic lithotrites (EHL) or mechanical impacters.

Routine swelling of the ureter is managed with a double-J stent, which decreases the risk of a blocked ureter and makes urinary drainage easier. This reduces flank pain and the risk of infection associated with an obstructed ureter. This stent is placed through the ureter via an endoscope under x-ray control.

Complications Ureteroscopy is a simple and straightforward procedure in the hands of a trained urologist, but there can be complications, as with any procedure.

◆ The ureter may be perforated, but if this is recognized early during treatment it is managed by inserting a double-J stent. If the stone has not been completely removed when the perforation is made, the ureteroscopy may have to be repeated.

◆ Ureteroscopic manipulation may dislodge the impacted stone back into the kidney, particularly if the ureter is dilated above the stone because of a long-standing obstruction. If the stone migrates too far back into the kidney to allow its removal by the ureteroscope, ESWL may be neces-

sary to complete treatment.

◆ These complications may cause constant severe loin pain for several weeks after treatment once the double-J stent has been removed.

◆ There is also a risk that urinary infections may become worse, although the risk is significantly reduced if antibiotics are given before the procedure.

After the Ureteroscopy Blood in the urine is normal after ureteroscopy, particularly if a double-J stent is in place because the stent may rub against the walls of the ureter and the bladder. Blood loss is minimal, yet even a few drops are enough to produce red, bloody urine. This usually subsides within 48 hours of the stent being removed. It is unusual for blood loss to be so significant as to form clots. If clots do appear, contact your urologist.

Double-J stents may produce symptoms of their own.

◆ You may feel burning or stinging with urination and the need to empty your bladder during the first few days the stent is in place.

◆ You may have flank pain during urination, as urine may be forced back into the kidney rather than discharging through the urethra. Interrupting the urinary stream will stop severe pain. Such symptoms usually subside after three or four days, as the plastic of the stent softens. After this time, you will usually be unaware that a stent is in place.

◆ Double-J stents always must be removed, because if they are left in place for too long, stones may form along the stent itself. Some stents have a string attached and are removed by a urologist pulling on the string. But removal is usually performed without a regional anesthetic, using a pair of small graspers passed through a telescope into the bladder. You may feel some discomfort, but the procedure is not usually painful.

SURGERY TO THE SCROTUM

After all surgical procedures to the scrotum, special attention has to be paid to rest and recuperation, pain control and the use of supportive dressings and underwear.

Surgical Procedure: Vasectomy The vas deferens is the small muscular tube that transmits sperm from the testicles to the prostate. Ligation, or the tying off, of the vas deferens prevents sperm from passing into the urinary tract and being ejaculated. A vasectomy, therefore, is permanent contraception for men.

A small incision is made in each side of the scrotum. The vas deferens is lifted through the wound and is cut and tied. Dissolvable sutures are usually used to close the wound. The stitches dissolve over four to six weeks, during which time you may notice some swelling and redness in the region.

After the Operation Rest at home for 24 hours after your vasectomy and avoid any heavy exertion.

♦ Exertion may cause significant bleeding from the vasectomy site, resulting in a large pool of blood collecting in the scrotum. If this happens, contact your urologist immediately.
♦ You may bathe in two or three days.
♦ You should wear a scrotal support or firm-fitting underwear for a week.
♦ There may be sperm in the vas deferens beyond the site where it is cut and tied, so normal fertility may persist for up to 12 ejaculations after the operation. Additional contraceptive procedures will be required during this time.
♦ Semen analysis will confirm the absence of sperm before you discontinue other forms of contraception.
♦ There will be no change in sexual sensation after the vasectomy. The seminal vesicles and prostate are unaffected, so you won't notice any change in the volume of the ejaculate.

Surgical Procedure: Hydrocele Repair About 5 to 10 percent of newborn boys have a collection of fluid around the testes called a hydrocele. The condition may also develop later in life.

An incision is made in the wall of the scrotum. The testis is lifted through, per-

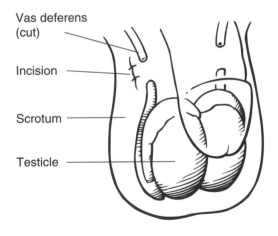

Vas deferens (cut)

Incision

Scrotum

Testicle

Vasectomy

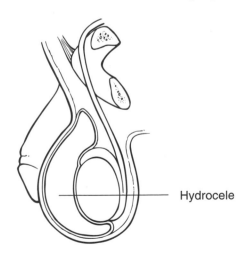

Hydrocele

Hydrocele

mitting the walls of the hydrocele to be cut and reconfigured so that the fluid collection will not recur. Dissolvable sutures are routinely used to close the wound.

After the Operation Rest is essential for several days after the operation to prevent bleeding.

◆ Dressings have to be worn over the wound, and the area has to be supported by firm-fitting underwear or a truss.

◆ Tylenol or other commercial medications are usually enough to manage pain. Drugs containing aspirin should not be taken, as they increase the likelihood of bleeding.

Surgical Procedure: Varicocele A varicocele is a collection of large dilated veins draining the testes, usually the left testicle. This may cause significant symptoms, including testicular pain and infertility.

Traditionally, a varicocele was repaired through a 2 to 3 in. (5 to 8 cm) incision made either in the groin or in the abdominal wall. The veins draining the testes were tied off, which meant they would gradually shrink, the pain would subside and the infertility would resolve. The testicles would then drain through numerous small veins that otherwise play a minimal role.

Repairing varicoceles this way is still routine, but new laparoscopic techniques allow treatment through smaller incisions in an attempt to reduce discomfort. One large incision may be much more painful than several smaller ones. With either open or laparoscopic techniques, the varicocele mass shrinks and the pain subsides over the first few weeks.

Surgical Procedure: Removing the Testicles (Orchiectomy) The testicles may have to be removed as part of the treatment for certain types of cancer. They are removed in two ways, depend-

ing on the condition being treated.

◆ If the orchiectomy is being done as part of the treatment for prostate cancer that has spread (metastatic), an incision will be made in the scrotum and the testicles removed. After the procedure, you will have to see your urologist on a regular basis indefinitely.

◆ Orchiectomy for cancer of the testes, usually seen in young men, is performed through an inguinal, or groin, incision. It is of particular importance that you rest quietly for several days after such a procedure and that you wear supportive garments and dressings.

Surgical Procedure: Undescended Testicles (Orchiopexy) Testicles that have not completely descended are not unusual in infant boys, particularly those born prematurely. If they have not descended into their normal position in the scrotum after 12 to 18 months, surgical placement of the testicles is usually warranted.

The condition often occurs in association with small hernias, which have to be repaired at the same time the testicles are brought down into the scrotum.

Small incisions are made in the groin. The testicles are usually cut free of the coverings that hold them in the abnormal position and secured in a small pouch made within the scrotum. Dissolvable sutures are used to close the incision.

After the Operation The procedure is usually well tolerated by young children, but the same considerations of care after scrotal surgery in adults apply.

◆ Pain is usually managed with a syrup form of paracetamol or acetaminophen.

◆ Care must be taken to keep the wounds clean and for your child to avoid unnecessary and strenuous activity during the first two weeks after surgery.

◆ Small bruises in the scrotal and groin regions are not uncommon.

◆ An expanding bulge caused by internal bleeding may have to be drained surgically, so notify your urologist immediately if a bulge appears.

SURGERY TO THE PENIS

Just as with scrotal surgery, care has to be taken after surgery to the penis. The need for rest and adequate pain control are paramount.

Surgical Procedure: Circumcision Circumcision is usually performed in children for religious purposes or for hygienic reasons. It is also performed in an adult as treatment for phimosis, a condition in which the foreskin can't be retracted over the shaft of the penis, preventing adequate hygiene. (figure 5).

The foreskin is excised in a circumferential fashion. Stitches bring together the cut edges of skin tissue about a third of the way down the shaft of the penis.

After the Operation It is normal to have normal daytime and nighttime erections after the operation. Not surprisingly, these are generally painful.

◆ Sexual intercourse should not be attempted for at least three or four weeks or until the surgical wound is well healed.

Surgical Procedure: Hypospadias Repair Hypospadias is a congenital condition in which the opening of the urethra, the meatus, occurs not on the tip of the penis but on the lower part of the shaft.

Repairing the condition usually involves rotating small flaps of skin from the sides of the penis to form a tube that elongates the urethra, which is then brought out in its normal position on the tip of the penis. A urethral stent may be inserted to ensure drainage of urine.

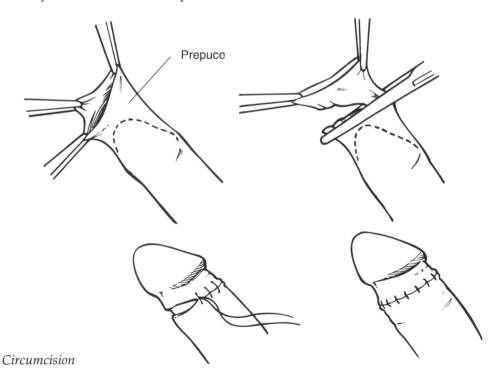

Circumcision

After the Operation Penile swelling and bruising are normal after the procedure. Your urologist should be contacted in cases of severe swelling, a high fever or poor urinary output.

QUESTIONS TO ASK YOUR UROLOGIST

◆ What type of anesthesia will be needed?

◆ What are the possible complications of the procedure?

◆ Will I have any catheters or tubes when I go home?

◆ Will I have to measure my urine output?

◆ Is blood in the urine to be expected?

◆ Will I have to restrict any of my activities after the operation?

◆ How long will the recovery period be?

GLOSSARY OF TERMS

A

Abscess
An undrained collection of pus anywhere in or on the body. Often appears as a red, hot, swollen lump that may be painful.

Ace wraps
Elasticized bandages used to wrap extremities to provide support for an area, help with circulation or reduce swelling.

Alkaline phosphatase
An enzyme released from the lining of the bile ducts that may be elevated with gallstone disease.

Allograft
A transplant of tissue from a healthy person who has died, usually from an injury. (*See also* Graft.)

Alopecia
Partial or complete loss of hair.

Anal condylomata
Skin outgrowths (tags) or warts found in the anal region.

Anal fissure
A split in the lining of the anal canal.

Anal fistula
A connection between the anal canal and the skin around the anus that causes intermittent pain, swelling and discharge.

Anesthesia, caudal
Regional anesthetic injected directly into the lower spinal canal.

Anesthesia, epidural
Regional anesthetic given continuously through a tube inserted near the nerves leading from the spinal column, causing numbness from the waist down.

Anesthesia, general
An anesthetic that numbs the whole body; the patient is unconscious. Given by injection or as a gas breathed in through a mask.

Anesthesia, local
An anesthetic injected directly into tissue to numb only the area to be operated on. Given with or without intravenous sedation.

Anesthesia, regional
An anesthetic that numbs an entire region of the body, such as an arm or both legs from the waist down. Given with or without intravenous sedation. Two common types are epidural and spinal.

Anesthesiologist
A medical doctor who specializes in the field of anesthesiology.

Anesthetic
A medication that causes loss of sensation.

Anesthetist
The person who administers the anesthetic. This person might be an anesthesiologist or a certified registered nurse anesthetist (CRNA).

Aneurysm
The stretching or dilation of the wall of an artery or vein.

Anorectal area
The final portion of the digestive tract, consisting of the rectum and anus. The rectum is the last 5 in. (12 cm) of the colon above the anus; the anus is the short muscular tube where the rectum opens to the body surface.

Anoscope
A short viewing tube used to examine the anal canal.

Anticoagulants
Substances such as aspirin or Coumadin that prevent blood from clotting. They are often stopped before elective surgery.

Anus
A 1 in. (2.5 cm) long muscular tube where the rectum opens to the body surface.

Appendix
A small, worm-like structure attached to the beginning of the large intestine, in the lower right abdomen.

Arteriogram
An x-ray procedure in which a dye is inject-

ed into an artery. The x-ray picture of arteries identifies blockages or dilated areas.

Arthroscope
A viewing tube used to examine the inside of a joint.

Arthroscopic surgery
Joint surgery performed with the aid of an arthroscope, which allows the surgeon to view what he or she is doing on a video screen.

Asymptomatic
Showing no symptoms.

Autologous blood
Your own blood used for a transfusion, given to a blood bank several weeks before the scheduled operation.

B

Bicoronal incision
An incision hidden in the hairline.

Biliary colic
Intense pain in the right upper abdomen, caused when a gallstone blocks the neck of the gallbladder.

Biopsy
The surgical removal of a small sample of tissue to determine a diagnosis.

Blepharoplasty
Surgery on the eyelids.

Bronchoscope
A viewing tube passed down the throat to examine the trachea (windpipe) and bronchi.

Brow ptosis
An anatomic deformity in which the eyebrow and its accompanying skin drop below the brow ridge because of lax muscles and softening tissues.

Bunions
Bony growths on the outside of the base of the big toe.

C

Cardiac monitor
A machine that assesses your heart rhythm during surgery.

Cataract
A clouding of the transparent lens of the eye.

Catheter
A thin rubber, plastic or metal tube inserted into a body cavity or vein to drain fluid or deliver fluids or medication.

Certified Registered Nurse Anesthetist
A CRNA is highly qualified to administer anesthesia.

Cholecystectomy
Removal of the gallbladder. This is the most common operation performed laparoscopically.

Cholecystitis
Inflammation of the gallbladder caused by the persistent blockage of the neck of the gallbladder by a gallstone.

Chronic
Pain, illness or disease that lasts a long time.

Circumcision
Removal of the foreskin of the penis.

Colonoscope
A long, flexible viewing tube used to examine the entire colon.

Colposcope
A viewing tube used to examine the vagina and cervix.

Cone biopsy
Removal of a small cone of abnormal cervical tissue with a scalpel or laser.

Conjunctiva
The thin mucous membrane covering the eyeball and lining the eyelids.

Cornea
A transparent membrane that forms the outer coat of the eyeball.

CT (computerized tomography) scan
An x-ray study that provides cross-section images of the inside of the body.

Cyst
A fluid-filled sac of tissue. Found in many parts of the body.

Cystectomy
Removal of a cyst.

Cystogram
An x-ray picture of the bladder.

Cystoscope
A viewing tube used to examine the inside of the bladder.

D

Deviated septum
A deviated septum results in obstructed airways. It is typically caused by a developmental problem or a history of injuries to the nose.

Dissection
The surgical cutting apart or separating of tissue.

Doppler ultrasound
Used to listen to the veins and arteries to acquire information about blood flow. (*See* Ultrasound.)

Drain
A small plastic tube used to drain fluid from a wound after surgery. It usually stays in place for about one week.

E

Ectopic pregnancy
Pregnancy that occurs when a fertilized egg, or ovum, implants anywhere outside the uterine cavity.

EKG (electrocardiogram)
A graph showing the heart's rhythm, obtained using an electrocardiograph machine.

Electrocauterization
The use of heat to seal blood vessels to stop bleeding.

Electrocoagulation
The use of an electric current to seal blood vessels to stop bleeding.

End-tidal carbon dioxide monitor
A device that measures the amount of carbon dioxide in your exhaled breath to give an accurate picture of your metabolic level.

Endometrial ablation
In this procedure, a "roller ball" instrument is inserted through a hysteroscope to burn (coagulate) the endometrial lining to stop endometrial bleeding.

Endometrial biopsy
A biopsy of the uterine lining.

Endometriosis
Endometrial implants outside the uterine cavity. These implants can be throughout the pelvic area and respond to hormonal cycles similar to the lining of the uterus. Most patients with endometriosis have painful menstrual cycles.

Endometrium
The lining of the uterus, shed each month during the menstrual cycle.

Endoscopy
Examination of organs or body cavities with a telescope-like viewing tube (endoscope). The surgeon can take photographs, obtain small samples of tissue or remove small growths during the procedure. (*See also individual scopes.*)

Excision
The surgical removal of tissue or an organ.

Extracorporeal shock waves (Lithotripsy)
Shock waves from an external source that pass through the body wall and disintegrate kidney stones.

F

Fascia
A thick, leathery layer of connective tissue, one of several layers of the abdominal wall.

Fluoroscopy
Examination of the inside of the body using live x-rays on a video screen. A fluoroscope is a machine that allows x-rays of a part of the body to be projected on a monitor so that it may be seen live during a procedure or operation.

Free-standing facility
An outpatient surgery facility that is not part of a hospital.

G

Gastroscope
A viewing tube passed down the throat to examine the inside of the stomach.

General anesthesia
See Anesthesia.

Glaucoma
A disease of the eye characterized by increased pressure inside the eyeball, which can result in damage to the optic disc and nerve fibers and interfere with vision.

Graft
Tissue transplanted from one part of the body to another. (*See also* Allograft.)

H

Hammer toes
Deformities of the four small toes, giving them a claw-like shape.

Hematoma
Bleeding and/or a collection of blood under the skin.

Hematuria
Blood in the urine.

Hemorrhoidectomy
Surgical removal of large hemorrhoids that protrude through the anus and don't respond to common therapy.

Hemorrhoids
Dilated veins beneath the lining of the anal canal. They may bleed, drop down from the rectum through the anus (prolapse), itch or develop blood clots (thrombose). Thrombosed hemorrhoids are swollen and painful. Treatment depends on the size and degree of inflammation and the degree of prolapse.

Hernia
An abnormal hole in the body through which internal organs can protrude.

Histology
Analysis of tissue under the microscope to determine a diagnosis.

Hydrocele
A collection of fluid around the testis.

Hypospadias
A congenital condition in which the opening of the urethra, the meatus, is not on the tip of the penis but on the lower part of the shaft.

Hysteroscope
A viewing tube used to examine the uterus.

I

Incision
A surgical cut.

Intravenous (IV)
Administering medications or fluids directly into a vein.

Intravesical chemotherapy
The delivery of chemotherapeutic drugs into the bladder through a catheter.

J

Jack-knife position
The patient lies face down on the operating table. The middle of the table is raised so that the hips are flexed, giving the surgeon access to the anorectal area.

K

Kidney dialysis
People whose kidneys fail to perform their main function of filtering fluid wastes from the blood have to have their blood purified by an artificial kidney, or hemodialysis machine.

L

Laparoscope
A small scope passed into the belly with a small camera attached, which a surgeon uses to view the abdominal organs.

Laparoscopic surgery
Surgery performed through small incisions; the surgeon's hands remain outside the patient's body. A tiny video camera is inserted through one incision so the surgeon can view the operative area on a video screen. Long, thin surgical instruments are inserted through other small incisions.

Laparoscopy
Examination of the pelvis and abdomen using an intra-abdominal telescope (laparoscope). This can help determine the cause of pelvic pain or determine tumor spread in prostate or bladder cancers.

Laparotomy
In an exploratory laparotomy, the abdomen is opened so the surgeon can explore the organs to find out what is wrong.

Laryngoscope
A viewing tube used to examine the larynx (voice box).

Liposuction
Removal of fat from areas of the body using suction. Also called fat suction or suction lipectomy.

Lithotomy position
The patient lies face up with legs spread and feet suspended in stirrups.

Lithotripsy
A standard treatment for kidney stones that uses sound waves to disintegrate the stones inside the body.

Long-term vascular access
The delivery of medication or other fluids directly into a vein through a small plastic tube called a catheter. This method is used when a patient must receive medication or other fluids for extended periods. This avoids the inconvenience and discomfort of frequent restarting of intravenous lines.

M

Metastasis
The spread of cancer from one part of the body to another by way of the lymph system or bloodstream.

MRI (magnetic resonance imaging)
A method of creating three-dimensional images of the inside of the body using a magnetic field and radio waves rather than x-rays.

N

Non-tunneled catheter
A catheter that enters the skin and the vein at the same place.

O

Occult blood
Hidden blood, usually in the stool, that can be detected only by special tests.

Oophorectomy
Removal of the ovary.

Orchiectomy
Removal of the testicles.

Orthopedics
The field of medicine concerned with correcting or curing diseases of the bones, joints and other parts of the skeletal system.

Orthostatic hypotension
A phenomenon in which the blood pressure decreases when you stand up from a sitting or reclining position.

Osteotomy
Cutting of the bone.

Outpatient surgery
The common term for when a patient arrives at a surgical suite in the morning, undergoes surgery, has a brief recovery, then goes home the same day. Also called ambulatory surgery or day surgery.

P

Pancreatitis
An inflammation of the pancreas. Often occurs when a gallstone blocks the duct draining the pancreas, which enters the intestine at the same point as the bile duct.

Pap smear
A screening test for precancer and cancer of the cervix in which cells from the cervix are obtained for microscopic examination.

Pelvic inflammatory disease (PID)
PID is caused by an infection in the uterus, tubes and/or ovaries. The most common infectious organisms are gonorrhea and chlamydia. The infection can cause tubal damage, abscesses and scars.

Percutaneous
A procedure performed completely through small incisions through the skin.

Peripheral vascular surgery
Surgery on the blood vessels of the neck and limbs.

Peritonitis
An acute inflammation of the peritoneum, the membrane lining the abdomen.

Phacoemulsifier
An ultrasonic microsurgical tool used to remove an eye cataract. It breaks a cataract into small particles that can be vacuumed away.

Phlebitis
An inflamed vein.

Polyp
A small mushroom-like growth protruding into the tunnel (lumen) of the colon or rectum.

Proctoscope
A viewing instrument used to examine the anus and rectum.

Prognosis
The prediction of the outcome of a disease or illness.

Prolapsed
An organ that has fallen out of its normal position.

Ptosis
Sagging of an organ or part of the body, such as an eyelid or breast.

Pulse oximeter
A device that fits over the fingertip and can read the amount of oxygen in the bloodstream.

R

Rectum
The last 5 in. (12 cm) of the colon above the anus.

Regional anesthesia
See Anesthesia.

Retina
The back of the eye, containing specialized sensory cells that detect light and send an image to the brain.

Rhinoplasty
Nasal surgery involving reshaping the nasal bones and/or the tip of the nose.

Rhytidectomy
A facelift operation.

S

Sedation
Being deeply relaxed or put to sleep by a medication (sedative).

Sigmoidoscope
A viewing tube used to examine the rectum and the portion of the colon immediately above the rectum (the Sigmoid colon). There are two basic types: rigid and flexible.

Sitz bath
Soaking the anorectal area in the bathtub or a shallow pan of warm water.

Skin tag
A polyp or small outgrowth of skin.

Speculum
An instrument for enlarging the opening of any canal or cavity to allow examination of its interior.

Stenosis
A narrowing of any canal or opening in the body.

Subcutaneous
Below the skin.

Suprapubic catheter
A catheter used to relieve the bladder of urine without having a catheter pass through the urethra. It usually enters the bladder through the skin just above the pubic bone and is connected to a standard catheter bag.

T

Tourniquet
A band or bandage tightened to slow or stop blood flow.

Trendelenburg position
The patient is tilted at a 45-degree angle, with the head and shoulders below knee level.

Trocar
An instrument used for withdrawing fluid from a cavity.

Tubal ligation
Sealing the fallopian tube – by coagulation or by placing a small ring to strangulate the tube – to block passage of sperm or ova.

Tunneled external catheter
A catheter that travels under the skin for several inches before it enters the vein.

U

Ultrasound
High-frequency sound waves emitted from a probe placed on the skin. The waves are reflected in varying intensities to produce an image of an organ on a video screen.

Ureteroscopy
The use of a high-pressure balloon to dilate the opening of the ureter as it enters the bladder. This eases the passage of a flexible scope used to extract large kidney stones or fragments.

Urethrogram
An x-ray procedure that produces an image of the urethra.

Urethroscope
A viewing instrument used to examine the urethra.

Urinary calculi
Urinary stones. They form in the collecting system of the kidney and may grow to a size of several inches.

Urodynamic profile
A test that evaluates the pressures produced in the bladder and in the urinary sphincter during urinating and at various levels of bladder filling.

V

Varicocele
A collection of large dilated veins draining the testes, usually the left testicle. This may cause significant symptoms, including testicular pain and infertility.

Varicose veins
Bulging, bluish veins on the legs. Caused when valves inside the veins that are supposed to keep blood flowing upwards toward the heart become defective and weak, allowing blood to flow backward.

Vas deferens
The secretory duct of the testicle through which semen travels during ejaculation. Ligation, or tying off, the vas deferens prevents sperm from passing into the urinary tract and being ejaculated.

Vasogram
X-ray contrast dye is injected into the vas deferens to detect any blockages between the testes and the urinary tract.

Venogram
The injection of dye through a small catheter inserted into a vein in the foot. The dye shows up on a series of x-rays taken of the veins and indicates narrowing, blockages or swelling of the veins.

Vital signs
Your temperature, pulse rate, respiratory (breathing) rate and blood pressure.

INDEX